# The: Smart Life Series: Couch to Health

## Sean Simonds, PT, DPT, OCS, CSCS

## 2015

## Other Resources

www.facebook.com/SmartLifeSeries ←Like us!

www.TheSmartLifeSeries.com

http://www.thesmartlifeseries.com/smart-life ←follow us

## Dedication

Thank you to my entire, wonderful family. With special thanks to my ever supportive parents and wife.

SMART LIFE™

## Education and Certifications

**2004-2006:** AFAA certified Personal Trainer

**2007:** B.S. from James Madison University in Kinesiology with a concentration in Exercise Science

**2009:** Earned strength and conditioning specialty (CSCS) from the National Strength and Conditioning Association (NSCA)

**2010:** Doctorate of Physical Therapy from St. Francis University

**2009-2010:** Clinical rotations in in-patient rehabilitation (Gavinana, Italy), pediatric oncology and adult stroke (Morgantown, WV), outpatient sport (Morgantown, WV) and orthopedics (Roanoke, VA).

**2001-2007, 2011-Present**: USSF certified Soccer Referee

**2010-2012**: Physical therapist/clinic manager at two private outpatient clinics in Virginia and PRN work at a rehab facility.

**2014:** Board Certified Orthopedic Clinical Specialist

**2015**: Owner of Specialized Physical Therapy of the Carolinas

# Table of Contents

# Introduction

*"The evolutionary record makes it clear that humans are born to be active." –Karen Steudel, PhD University of Wisconsin-Madison*

*Initial Information*

Age: _____          Height: _____          BMI: _____

Weight: _____          Heart Rate: _____          % Body Fat: _____

Blood Pressure: _____          Total Cholesterol: _____

Waist Size: _____          Are you healthy? _____

*Purpose*

The purpose of this book is simple—**to help you live a healthy lifestyle.** This book outlines a process covering an entire year. Before closing the book and scoffing at "one year" and #gettinghealthysucks, give it a chance. Unfortunately, there is no magic pill to living healthy. Anyone that tries to convince you otherwise is <u>lying</u>. If it were true, that person would be the richest and most popular person ever. The fact is most people who make drastic changes over night are unable to maintain these for any significant amount of time. Eventually, you are back where you started (or worse in most cases). This is why fad diets are extremely efficient initially, but fail in the long run. This book will carefully guide you month-by-month through a complete lifestyle change. Progress will be gradual and lasting. It is my hope that, by the end of the year you will be better educated on health and wellness and that you will be a **healthier and happier person**. This book will not promote a get fit quick or lose weight today scheme of any kind. If that is what you are looking for, you might as well close the book.

The program I have developed is presented in a simple manner with a lot of areas for you to record and participate. The plan is supposed to cover most areas of a healthy lifestyle. I will cover diet, exercise, motivation, overall wellness, goals/rewards, etc. I am hoping that this will provide you with all of the tools you need to make these changes and be successful long-term.

Each chapter will provide you with information, tips and strategies, new goals, and new changes/additions to your life. In order for everything to work, these changes/additions to your life must be kept and carried over from month to month so they become part of your every day life, for the rest of your life. If in one month you walk 20 min/day, you should walk 20 min/day everyday from then on (if this is your goal).

Each major topic will be introduced twice. The first time will have a little background and some changes to be made. Then a few months down the road, this same topic will be revisited and you will have the opportunity to expand on these goals and take them to the next level. It is important to point out that you are in control of these goals. I will make suggestions based on things I have done and seen, but ultimately, it will be up to you. Make sure to participate, as it will only improve your experience and your chance for success.

The book is called "Couch to Health" but the principles discussed throughout this book can be applied to people of all levels of health. Pointers will be thrown in for the more advanced exerciser as we go along.

*Some Background...*

The chart on the next page is showing the major categories (at least in the eyes of the author) contributing to overall health and wellness. Think about what makes you healthy in all aspects of life. Try and come up with a goal for each!

What does your chart look like?  What is important to you?

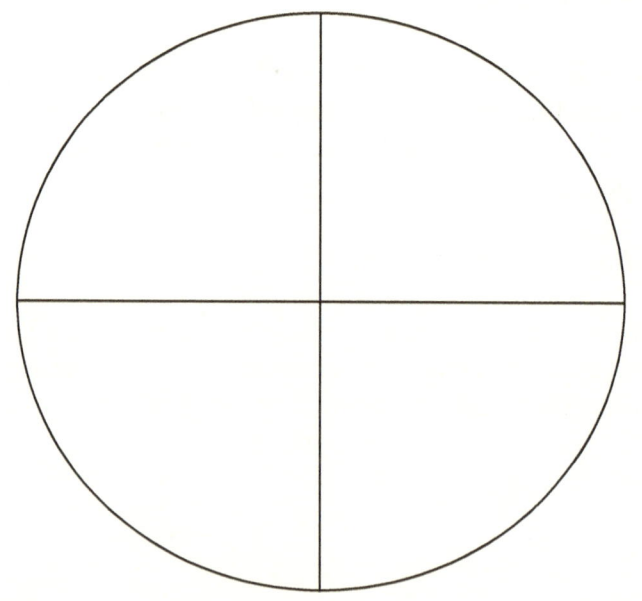

Before we get into things, please complete the goal list below. The idea is to come up with goals you hope to accomplish by the end of this program. I have provided examples of my goals I chose when I started this (yes, I followed the program to make sure it was useful and worked). Feel free to incorporate short and long-term goals. It is the intent of this book to pay attention to all aspects of your health.

My sample goal list:
1. Incorporate 30 min of cardio and 30 min of resistance training on 5/7 days/week.
2. Lower my blood cholesterol to 140 (total).
3. Have more energy and feel more relaxed at the end of long days.

Your goal list. What you hope to change or achieve.
1. _____
2. _____
3. _____
4. _____
5. _____
6. _____
7. _____
8. _____
9. _____
10. _____

**In the space below insert a picture of yourself.**

*Quality of Life and Healthy Years*

This is what it is all about. Quality of Life is one of the most important aspects of losing weight and living a healthier lifestyle. Basically, you want to be able to do the activities you enjoy without poor health getting in the way. Being healthy allows you to interact with your environment and maintain your independence.


Health should not be considered the absence of illness. I ask all my patients do you think you are generally healthy? So many times I get, "Yes. I've only been sick enough twice in my life to go see a doctor." Yet, the person sitting in front of me is overweight with arthritic knees and back that cannot walk for more than 3 minutes without pain. Health needs to be seen as a much more global concept. The CDC states that, "Health is optimal well-being that contributes to one's quality of life. Optimal health includes high-level mental, social, emotional, spiritual, and physical wellness within the limits of one's heredity and personal abilities." Basically, there are many parts that make up a healthy lifestyle and all must be addressed to be truly healthy.

Ask yourself right now. "Am I healthy?" What are your answers (comment below!)? Are you overweight? Do you have diabetes? Do you get out of breath with minimal exertion? How far can you walk/jog/run? Does anything limit these activities? What do you do for fun? Is there any activity that you want to do that you can't because you aren't physically able?




What does it mean to you to be healthy?

Let's get back to the pie chart. Has anything changed?

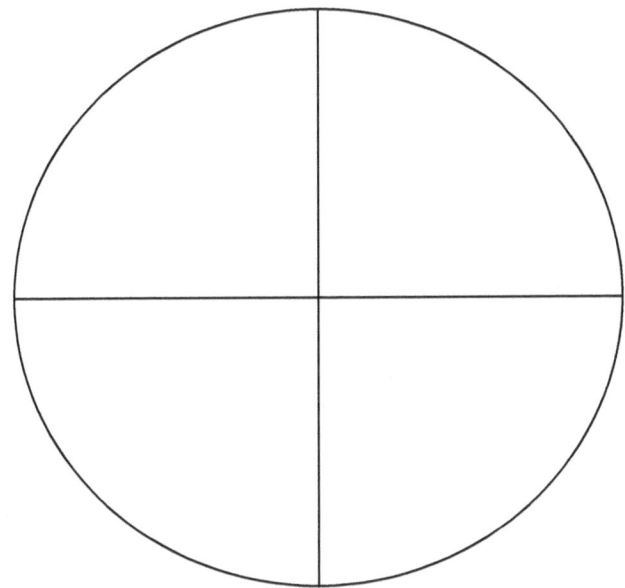

Other things people have showed me in their pie charts:
1. Personal growth and spirituality
2. Movement
3. Nutrition
4. Relationships
5. Interaction with the environment
6. Access to quality Physical Therapists, Nutritionists, Strength and conditioning specialists

What about your goals now? Have they changed?
1. _____
2. _____
3. _____
4. _____


*Wellness*

"A well person is satisfied in work, is spiritually fulfilled, enjoys leisure time, is physically fit, is socially involved, and has a positive emotional-mental outlook." --JMU Lifetime Fitness and Wellness

Research supports the idea that a person's self-perception of wellness are more important than actual ability. This is great news because very few of us can run ultra-marathons or score under-par at most golf courses, but most of us can be perfectly happy jogging along a path for a couple miles and enjoy the experience.

The concepts of health and wellness go together. Eating healthy foods and staying physically fit are great but can actually harm your quality of life if you are miserable all the time. This is why we will be making small changes throughout this process and not wholesale changes on day one. If you start a diet that says, "no more steak, ever again" and you like steak, put the book down and move on. The goal with all of this is to make you healthy **and** happy. Here is something really cool to keep in mind. A lot of people say they don't like to exercise. But ask them sometime how they feel after exercise and you might get a different answer. The reason you should do this is because exercise releases powerful "feel good" chemicals in your body. Exercise has been shown to improve mood, decrease stress, decrease blood pressure, and make you feel better in general.

All of this comes back to quality of life. To have a high quality of life you should be able to do enjoyable things with little or no limitations. We want to improve **quality** of life.

Remember that this healthy lifestyle we are supporting here is also meant to reduce your risk of other problems. Regular physical activity and a healthy diet help reduce the risk of heart disease, stroke, type 2 diabetes, obesity, high blood pressure, colon caner, and early death. When you look at the seriousness of these diseases, exercise and healthy eating seem like such an easy sacrifice to make!

Todays task--Answer the following questions on a piece of paper. When you are having a tough time motivating yourself to exercise or eat healthy, look at your answers.

1. What makes you happy?

2. What do you hope to achieve by starting this healthy lifestyle?

3. Who are you doing this for?

*Daily Activity*

There are many studies and surveys out there that look at how much exercise people used to get and how much they do now. One study on Amish men showed that they averaged more than 10hrs of vigorous activity and 43hrs of moderate activity each week! Todays Americans might walk a mighty 5,000 steps a day (which is almost nothing).

Fortunately, the benefits of exercise come almost immediately after starting even a modest level of activity. Many people are credited for saying, "Getting off the couch conveys the greatest results." This just means that going from nothing to something yields the most significant benefits.

In the book, "The First 20 Minutes," a study out of the University of Cambridge was noted. Their results stated "a person's risk of dying prematurely from any cause plummeted nearly 20 percent if he or she began to meet the current exercise guidelines of 150 minutes of moderate activity per week." It is a far cry from the numbers put up by Amish men, but it is enough to see significant health benefits.

The point is... Get up and get moving!

The American College of Sports Medicine (ACSM) has just released new recommendations on the quantity and quality of exercise for adults, definitively answering the age-old question of how much exercise is actually enough.

The following is pulled directly from the ACSM website:

The position stand, titled "Quantity and Quality of Exercise for Developing and Maintaining Cardiorespiratory, Musculoskeletal, and Neuromotor Fitness in Apparently Healthy Adults: Guidance for Prescribing Exercise," reflects current scientific evidence on physical activity and includes recommendations on aerobic exercise, strength training and flexibility. Consistent with the 2008 Physical Activity Guidelines for Americans, ACSM's overall recommendation is for most adults to engage in at least 150 minutes of moderate-intensity exercise each week.

"The scientific evidence we reviewed is indisputable," said Carol Ewing Garber, Ph.D., FAHA, FACSM, chair of the writing committee. "When it comes to exercise, the benefits far outweigh the risks. A program of regular exercise – beyond activities of daily living – is essential for most adults."

*Metabolic Fitness*

It is important to keep in mind throughout fitness routine that weight loss is not the only goal. It is very important to a lot of people starting a routine like this, but there are many good things that also happen including, but not limited to:

- decreased blood pressure and heart rate
- decreased fat and cholesterol levels in the blood
- better regulation of blood sugars
- improved bone density

Everyone can benefit from a healthy lifestyle program. Everyone can see improvement. No matter how far gone you are you can always get benefit out of healthy eating and exercise.

I'm telling you all this because most people want to make healthy changes to their lives but, in the end, fail to follow through for one reason or another. Most people get discouraged that they aren't losing weight fast enough or they don't see enough improvement in muscle definition and just stop. Remember that when you are active, improvements **are** occurring whether you can see them right away or not.

A handy little tool is a heart rate monitor. Amazon has some good ones for about $60. This can show you your heart rate in real time. It is great feedback and reinforcement to see your heart rate during exercise. On day 1, wear it while you work out and note the highest number it gets to. Then, in 4 weeks, do an identical workout and prepare to be amazed that your heart rate is lower throughout the routine! Seeing your heart rate go from 80 beats per minute to 70 or 60 beats per minute might not seem all that exciting. It certainly doesn't make you look any better in a bathing suit, right? But it is a wonderful indicator of how hard your heart is working. We want your hear to be lean and efficient at getting blood and nutrients to your body. As your heart rate drops it is showing that your heart has to work less to pump the same amount of blood. Example: On day 1 you run up that terrible hill near your house and your heart rate gets up to 120. In a month you run the same hill and your heart only gets up to 110. This means your heart had to beat 10 less times to perform the same activity. Add this up over a lifetime and you can really save your heart from a lot of work. Trust me, your heart appreciates it.

This is all a long way of saying; don't get too bogged down by the number on the scale in the bathroom. There are many other numbers that you want to change too!

*Adherence*

As you gear up for this new healthy lifestyle have you thought about how you will maintain this? It is a lifestyle change that you want to carry on forever. Various research reports that approx. 50% of all people who start a program like this will drop out within 6 months. A lot of the dropouts are due to poor planning. Here are a few tips to help you prepare.

1. **Decide where most of your workouts will occur.** Many dropouts are due to exercise becoming "inconvenient." If your gym is 45min away, you are setting yourself up for failure. Find somewhere close to exercise. It can be your home, a gym, the field out back, anything. Just make sure it is convenient.

2. **Make sure your first few workouts are relatively brief and manageable.** Some people don't like how exercise feels initially. Starting slow and gradually working your way up to longer and more intense workouts is a smart way to go.

3. **Have attainable short and long-term goals.** For example: "I will exercise 30minutes, 4x this week." OR "I will walk 1 mile 5x this week." I will run my first 5K in 3 months. Set them up so you are achieving goals regularly.

4. **On those days where you just don't want to move, make sure you do a little.** Do something like 10 squats, 10 biceps curls, and walk 1/4 mile. That way you are doing something and most times if you can get started, you will do the whole workout.

5. **Variety.** This is the most important one for me. I get bored quickly. If I did the same exact routine every week for 6 months, I'd never exercise. Try new things. Add some flavor to your routines.
Sample Week:
Monday: weight lifting for legs, bike for cardio
Tuesday: Rock climbing gym for arms, walked for cardio
Wednesday: Rest
Thursday: weight lifting for arms, bike for cardio
Friday: did exercise machine circuit training at the gym
Saturday: swam at the pool
Sunday: hiked
That is a lot of variety for one week, but you get the idea. People who do the exact same thing each week/month/year usually end up getting bored and quitting.

6. **Gym selfies are not cool.** BUT, getting people involved in this lifestyle change of yours IS cool. Starting with a physical therapist so you know what to do and how to do it safely is a great idea. Then get your spouse, kids, or friends involved. Find a gym buddy. Join an exercise class. I have a patient who is not a fan of exercising and I gave her this advice and her response was, "Why? Because misery loves company?" Maybe, but finding a gym buddy makes it more fun and makes you more accountable.

7. **Finally, monitor your progress.** This is where starting with a physical therapist is a great idea. You can always go back to them for "check ups" to monitor your gains. A lot of people like keeping an exercise journal, blog, or pinterest page, which are all great ideas. Have something definitive to look at so you know you are making progress. Make sure to at least track the things that are important to you.

All of the concepts covered in this first section will be revisited throughout the program.

Each month will start with a goal. The goals are pretty vague in some cases. This is on purpose so you can tailor it to your needs. It is important to achieve the goal each month before moving on to the next month. These goals are meant to build on each other.

Are you ready? Time to get to work.

# Month 1: Planning stage

*Goal: Prepare and organize your life to allow you to begin your lifestyle change. Buy a calendar or notebook to write everything down in or learn how to use the calendar on your smart phone to get started.*

The fact that you have this book means that you are at least contemplating getting started, and maybe you have even begun this journey and are looking for guidance. In either case, I can help.

The first thing you will notice reading this chapter is that there are no recommended changes to your diet, exercise, etc. It is true; this chapter (and much of the next) is all about planning and setting you up for success. These are the stages that never get enough attention and which ultimately lead to people not maintaining their life changes. These stages tend to be skipped. Most people will stand on a scale or get invited to the beach and realize that they have let themselves go. Looking at the extra insulation around their midsection, they think, "Oh shit." Now it is crunch time and they have to lose weight and get looking good fast. No planning or preparation is done and as soon as that beach weekend is over, their lives go right back to normal until the cycle starts all over. This stage is crucial and will allow you to smoothly move through the months ahead with minimal distractions. If you need an extra month, this is the place to take it. You need a solid foundation to set yourself up for success.

In the mean time you should not just sit on the couch and watch hours of re-runs you did not like the first time. As part of this planning month, you need to figure out what you like to do. Try new exercises, foods, and sources of motivation (even if it is just one time). Here are just a few suggestions:

☙

*Cardio*: stationary biking, mountain biking, hiking, rock climbing, rowing, kayaking, walking, jogging, running, swimming, zoomba, jazzercise, etc.

*Resistance Training*: free weights, machine weights, suspension bands, rubber bands, body weight, pulley systems, kettle bells, medicine balls, circuit training, etc

*Flexibility*: yoga, pilates, static stretching, dynamic stretching, tai chi, etc

*Diet*: strawberries, melons, whole grains, spinach, nuts, low fat/fat-free options, yogurt, peaches, raspberries, honeydew, chia seeds, flax seeds, quinoa, multi-grain, etc

*Motivation/Rewards*: food, movies, clothes, intrinsic, concerts, family, etc.

❦

These are widely known concepts in the exercise world that I am finding are more and more important for people to identify for themselves. Where you are on this continuum can greatly influence how you should approach exercise in order to make a permanent change.

The stages are:
1. ***Pre-contemplation:*** "I don't want to make a change."
2. ***Contemplation:*** "I am thinking about making a change."
3. ***Preparation:*** " I am getting ready to make a lifestyle change."
4. ***Action:*** "I have made some lifestyle changes."
5. ***Maintenance:*** "I regularly practice healthy lifestyle activities."

Maintenance should be what we all strive to achieve. But keep in mind that this is a continuum and you can move in either direction multiple times.

In-depth explanation below.....

Pre-contemplation
The good news is that you are already past this point just by reading this book. If you are reading this, you are at least a little interested in making a change. Congrats. Step 1 is complete.

Contemplation
"I am thinking about making a change."
Good. Sometimes just getting into that mindset that exercise is important can be the hardest part. If this is you, my suggestion is to continue doing some more research. Find out what exercise does for your body. Figure out why it usually ends up being a financial good decision. Discover why you'll live longer and feel better. Find out why it reduces stress and risk of stroke. Exercise is powerful stuff.

Preparation
This is the most skipped over part of this whole continuum, BUT the most important. People flirt with Action while sitting in the preparation phase. The biggest thing preventing you from moving into action and maintenance are roadblocks. Common roadblocks are: not enough time, don't like the exercises, cost, lack of motivation, etc. These roadblocks can prevent you from ever attaining maintenance. Preparation is the stage where you can clear all the roadblocks.

First, identify your potential roadblocks. Write them down and describe (briefly or extensively) each problem and why it is a problem. Then brainstorm potential solutions.

 Roadblocks are the primary reason healthy lifestyles don't stick.

For example, if you identify "time" as a potential roadblock as nearly 90% of Americans will identify, try writing out your schedule and then prioritizing the activities in the schedule. Another way to do it is look at activities that you can multi-task. *I had a patient* that was a parent with a daughter who had soccer practice 45 minutes away so she would stay for the 90 minute practice and sit in her car "looking up things" on her smartphone. We developed a 60 minute routine with exercise bands and 1 medicine ball that she could do easily while waiting for her daughter and still have time to play with her phone.

What are some roadblocks that you can see? How can you eliminate those? Write down each roadblock and strategize how to get rid of each.

1.

2.

3.

4.

5.

6.

7.

8.

9.

10.

Do not blow-off this step. Identifying all potential roadblocks and problem solving for them will greatly improve your odds at succeeding in this lifetime of health.

Next, find out what you like and where you like to do it. Do you like being around lots of people? Is going to a gym or working out at home better for you? Is the gym too expensive or is buying the necessary equipment to exercise at home going to be more costly?

Does cross-fit look interesting?  Or is working out with machines more your speed?  Try new things.  Most gyms will give you a couple visits to try it out.  Take advantage of this.  See what you like and what you hate.  There are many types of gyms.  They come in all sizes, offer a variety of equipment, costs, hours of operation, # of people, etc.

## Action
Congrats.  You are now making changes.  I have 2 simple tips for this stage.
1. Reassess, address, and eliminate any old or new roadblocks.
2. Plan ahead.  Make sure you know where you are going and how to get there.

Is a gym membership still in your budget?  How is the timing working out?  How often are you exercising these days?  Can you do more?

Setting goals helps you get from this stage to the next.  Plan to complete your first 5K.  It will require daily exercise and you will have a goal to fight for.

## Maintenance
One word.  VARIETY.  The quickest way to drop out of this is getting bored with the routine.  Change it up!  Find friends, switch gyms, try new routines, get a personal trainer, visit a physical therapist, and try a boot camp.  Don't let yourself get in a rut.

*Planning Your Exercise*

What do you think you need to do to get started?
1. _____
2. _____
3. _____
4. _____
5. _____

*Time*

Time is by far the primary reason for not starting and/or quitting a new routine. The bottom line is that no one has time. Everyone is always strapped for time. You can be a doctor on-call every night, a CEO of a major corporation, a student, or a retiree, no one has time. It is the people who **want to change** that are able to "find time." Sometimes it can be hidden and you just need to find it, other times it has to be created. If you look at your life and still cannot find even a second of time for physical activity (which many people swear is the case), then you are not looking and/or you do not actually want to make changes. I heard a friend complaining about not being able to find time in their schedule to exercise to which my best friend replied, "Does having a stroke and type II diabetes fit better into your schedule?" A joke, but unhealthy lifestyles, no exercise, stress, and poor diet, have caused a serious health epidemic in this country and the world. Obesity is linked to an enormous list of health problems, increasing healthcare costs for everyone, and premature, preventable death. The great thing about making calculated changes to your lifestyle is that we are not looking to make enormous time commitments. Our goal is to create a lifestyle that suits you and reduces your health risks.

A very common goal I tell friends and patients who are not used to regular exercise is to start with 15 min/day of walking. It seems simple enough right? Most people struggle to find 15 min/day where they can put everything down and just walk. It is a relatively easy exercise to start with whether you have exercised before or not. I suggest it to you right now. It does not matter if you have a treadmill, a walking path, or you just walk around the outside of your house for 15 min/day, you just have to do it. The great thing about the benefits of physical activity is that they do not have to be done in large chunks. The American College of Sports

Medicine and the American Heart Association recommend a total of 30 min/day of moderate physical activity. I am just asking for 15 min of walking. I had a patient recently tell me that she could not fit that into her day. I asked her to record what she did every minute of her day.

6:10am—7: alarm, prepared for work.
7—7:30: drove to work.
8—12: worked
12—1: sat in kitchen with lunch
1—1:10: waited for friend to go to meeting
1:10—3: meeting
3—5: worked at desk
5—5:45: drove home
5:45—7: got changed, made dinner, ate dinner
7—8: paperwork
8—10: TV
Bed

This is a typical day for most people working an 8—5 or 9—5 job. I found at least 6 time slots where a minimum of 5 minutes of walking could have gone. She could set her alarm 5 minutes early and do a quick walk before her morning shower. 5+ minutes could have been done at lunch and waiting for her friend after lunch. After getting changed and before dinner there are easily 5 minutes. Finally, 2 hours of TV time can be used much more productively. At the very least she could stand up and do a lap around her house during some of the commercial time. I suggested these simple adjustments to her schedule and she now walks 20-30 min/day.

**Time you didn't know existed**

1. Most people sit while talking on the phone. Stand up and walk around.
2. People sit at their desk at work all day. Rather than checking your email, walk around for a few minutes as your break.
3. Another surprising time is when you are brushing your teeth. Instead of sitting in front of a mirror, wander around the house for the entire time it takes to brush your teeth.

4. Take the stairs instead of the elevator/escalator.

 You do not need to block one and two-hour portions of your day off for exercise, especially when you are just getting started! 5 minutes here and there is a great way to start.

Once getting 15 minutes of walking in has become easy, try introducing and extra 5 minutes of something else (stretching, weights, etc.). You do not have to get sweaty and worn out for physical activity to be beneficial.

What are some times in your day you can sneak 5 min in? Do not make excuses, make the time.
1. _____
2. _____
3. _____

Eventually, you won't have to "sneak in" 5 minutes. A healthy lifestyle will just be what you do. You will exercise regularly, eat healthy, and interact with your environment positively. This healthy lifestyle change is not just about squeezing in a couple healthy habits; it is about making your life healthy. Look at your daily, weekly, and monthly routines. Strategize how you can better organize them to allow for this healthy lifestyle. Eventually, there should be a 1-hour scheduled time for exercise most days of the week.

*Creating a Supportive Environment*

Environments are tricky. Depending on where and who you live with, you can be in very different situations. The goal here will be making the most of your environment.

If it is just you and your spouse, there are a number of things you can try. Ask your spouse to get involved. Explain to them why this is beneficial to both of you and how important it is to you to have them involved. If they still do not want to, be strong and remember your goals. A lot of times if your spouse sees you motivated and actively improving your own life, they will be interested/motivated to join.

Use your exercise time as "together time." Most couples find it hard to fit in something as simple as talking to each other. Going for a walk around the block after work each day is great physical activity and allows 5-30 min/day of time to reconnect.

Avoid using guilt as a tool to get the stubborn spouse involved. It might seem like a great idea (I have tried it and failed), but your spouse will just grow to hate the activities.

*Physical Activity for You and Your Spouse*

Circuit training is a fast paced, ever changing style to try. Set up five stations. At each station, have a simple exercise set up (for example—walking, jumping jacks, bicep curls, sit-ups, squats). Set the timer for 3 minutes. Each of you is at a different station. Perform the physical activity, and then rotate to the next station when the 3 minutes is up.

**Radom Circuit**

| | | |
|---|---|---|
| A: squats | B: triceps pushes | C: chin-ups |
| D: Bike | E: Shoulder External Rotation | |

**Cardio Circuit**

| | | |
|---|---|---|
| A: Bike | B: Elliptical | C: Stepper |
| D: Rowing Machine | E: Treadmill | |

Team stretching is used in a lot of middle and high school sports. You stretch the other person's hamstrings for 5 minutes, then switch. Alternate as many times as you need to or have time for.

Long walks are a relaxing way to spend time with your spouse. Take your spouse (and pet) on a walk around the neighborhood or development.

Like we said before, not all spouses want to do some new physical activity. That's OK. Healthy lifestyle changes are **not** just physical activity. A lot of couples take up cooking healthy meals together. It can be used as time to talk about your day, watch a show, and just enjoy each other's company.

What lifestyle changes can you get your spouse involved in?

*Children*

Kids are a major obstacle for most parents trying to achieve a healthy lifestyle. Depending on the age, these obstacles will vary greatly. Very small children need constant attention. If your kid likes being held, pick them up and walk around the house/apartment for 5-10 min at a time. Do not just sit with them in your lap. Move with them! Rather than sitting on the couch making sure they do not do anything stupid (all children have the inherent desire to try and kill themselves), get down and roll around on the floor with them. Join in on their activities; you would be amazed at how hard it is to keep up with them! There was a fitness guru many years ago that decided to mimic a baby's movements for a whole day. He was unable to! It is a powerful mixture of isometrics, yoga, and static poses. Play with your child on the ground in a plank position or lie on your back and do 20 bridges.

What activities can you do with your small children?
1. _____
2. _____
3. _____

**Road Block Warning**
Children are a roadblock. Plain and simple. Take the time now to think about your child's needs, what they like doing, when/if you have any time to yourself. Write it in the space provided and then think about how you can get through it.
Ex. "My child wants to be held all the time."
Solution. Do 10 squats, switch the baby to the other hip, do 10 more. This can be done with most leg exercises.

Teenagers require you to become their personal taxi service at times. While you are sitting waiting for them, as you inevitably will, go for a short walk around their school (inside or out). I have a friend that has a couple of dumbbells in her car that she curls as she walks at her kid's baseball practice. Those 5, 10, 15 minutes waiting for your kids do not have to be wasted. Teenagers tend to create a lot of stress, especially for the caring parent. Physical activity is a great way to reduce teenager-related stress.

What activities can you do while waiting around for your teenager?
1. _____
2. _____
3. _____

Are there activities you and your teenager can do together?
Hiking, biking, cooking, going to the gym?

*The Home*

Make your home work. There is nothing to say that you have to walk 15 min around a track or on a path. My grandmother has a winding course through her house that takes her all of 45 sec -1 min to complete. She will do this for the 10 min and then rest. Use the long hallways, stairs, and hills on your property and in your home to your advantage. You may be required to tidy up around your house to clear walk-able paths. Is there a spare room that is the "junk" room? Can it be cleared and used as the new exercise room?

What are some ways you can improve your environment?
1. _____
2. _____
3. _____

Which room in your home can be used for exercise?

Do you have the necessary cooking supplies to make healthy meals?

Is there a place that is "your place" that you can go a unwind?

*Company*

Working out alone is boring (for most). Try and involve friends and family into your routine. You can include different people throughout the day. Walk with your spouse for 10 min before work, a friend for 10 min at lunch, and a neighbor for 10 min after work. Be creative. People tend to be more successful and more motivated when they are exercising with someone. If you do this routinely it adds accountability which can be very powerful.

Who are some friends/co-workers that you can involve? Which part of a healthy lifestyle can they be a part of?

1. _____
2. _____
3. _____
4. _____
5. _____

Ex. Joe—cooking class, Mary—Boot camp, Mike—book club

*Gym vs. Home*

**Roadblock Warning**
A lot of people get here, decide all this is going to be too expensive, and then stop. Do your research. An exercise routine can be done on almost any budget.

Will you do better in a gym, creating a home gym, or going to both? Here are some things to keep in mind when choosing or deciding to do a combination.

*Gym*
1. You will be around other people.
2. There is usually music playing.
3. Most places offer classes.
4. There is a lot of equipment.
5. Can be expensive.
6. Can have contracts.

7.   Motivates a lot of people to workout harder when there are people around.

*Home Gym*
1.   Exercise alone or with 1 or 2 select people.
2.   You choose the music or TV.
3.   On your schedule.
4.   Can be expensive to get enough equipment that you don't get bored.
5.   Easy to make excuses and skip a day.
6.   More comfortable.

The rest page is left blank to allow you to do a Pro's and Con's for each to help you decide which one, or a combo, is best suited for your needs.

For those who need to get out of the house and be around other people, the gym is great. The gym offers motivation, competition, people to talk to, guidance, advice, etc. Some businesses offer discounts at local gyms. Insurance companies are starting to reward their participants for daily exercise with reductions in insurance premiums and/or gym memberships. Contact your employer and insurance company to see what type of offers they provide. Some businesses have gyms in the building to encourage employees to exercise (exercise during the day has been shown to improve productivity and employee satisfaction, less days missed of work)→use them! Shop for the right gym for you. Cost, size, and services vary widely. Do your research. A good gym can be worth its weight in gold.

If your business and insurance company do not offer deals, it is time to shop around at local gyms.

What do you want in your gym?
1. _____
2. _____
3. _____
4. _____
5. _____

| My responses: | |
|---|---|
| 1. Budget friendly membership fee | 3. Basketball court |
| | 4. Good group classes |
| 2. Treadmills/elliptical | 5. Convenient hours |

Take this list of 5 things and find the gym that best meets your criteria. There are many gym-chains that are available in most places. Make sure you are getting what you want. If you do not, tell them you are taking your business elsewhere.

# Top 10 Questions to ask before signing a gym membership

1. Do you run promotional offers (reduction in membership cost)? I work at a local business, are there any deals for that? Is there a special family rate?
2. A lot of places will waive the "sign-up" fee. Do you?
3. How long is the membership for? What is the penalty if I decide to discontinue my membership before that time?
4. What are your normal business hours?
5. What are your rules regarding guests? Free passes? How many?
6. What classes are offered (and how often)? Is the price included in my membership?
7. Is the gym/pool used by other groups (local sports teams, high schools, etc)? When? Are the basketball courts closed at any other times?
8. Do you have personal trainers on staff? Does it cost extra to utilize their services (personal trainers, strength and conditioning specialists, athletic trainers, certified weight trainers)?
9. Are there times in the day where the equipment is full? Are there waits for machines?
10. What is your newest equipment? Do you have any "trendy" equipment (ie. Kettle bells, suspension bands, etc)?

*Home Gym*

If you are going to be splashing the cash on a gym membership, I do not personally see the need to have a full arsenal of work-out equipment in your home. If you go to the gym most days of the week, your equipment at home will become furniture, not workout equipment. However, if you are someone who will not be joining a gym, investing in some equipment for home will allow you to perform a wider variety of exercises and even provide some motivation. Working out at home can act as a stepping-stone for working out at the gym. I would suggest starting small with equipment. Getting some dumbbells of varying weights is a great start and will allow you to do a wide variety of weight training. A soft mat (yoga mat) is a smart purchase to make floor activities more comfortable. Suspension bands are a new piece of exercise equipment that offers a wide variety of whole body exercises. Exercise balls are becoming popular again for core strengthening. They are relatively cheap and help provide some variety to your routine.

| Equipment | Total |
|---|---|
| Yoga Mat, 20 lb kettle bell, suspension bands, exercise ball, glider (small rowing machine) | $35 + $35 + $50 + $20 + $145 = $285 for life! |
| Gym Membership | Month ($30-50)/Year ($360-600) |

What equipment do you think you will need?
1. _____
2. _____
3. _____
4. _____
5. _____

*Clothing*

Most people think you need designer workout clothes just to walk around a track at the gym. If you are a person that needs that, put it in your budget. Most people will be able to get away with an old pair of shorts (or sweats), a t-shirt, and sneakers. It is really that simple. Do not make it harder (or more expensive) than it needs to be. The one piece of clothing I would suggest investing in are your sneakers. They are extremely important for your comfort if you will be doing anything on your feet. Most local shoe stores (and even magazines) will have someone you can talk to about the right shoe for your body type and expected level of activity. I see people every week with injuries and/or pain from improper footwear. These aches and pains serve as an easy excuse not to exercise "just today" or "just this week". Do not fall into the trap! A pair of shoes is the one piece of attire worth spending money on.

Minimalist shoes are the new fad. I see people every week with stress fractures in their feet from running in them. My hope is that they fade like every other fad. My suggestion is to find a supportive, well-cushioned shoe to protect your feet.

> **Disclaimer:** *I am not a nutritionist or a dietician, nor do I pretend to be. All of the diet information given throughout this book are lifestyle recommendations. In other words, these diet tips are not targeted for any specific population. They are not made to lose weight, help with any specific disease, or any other problem. The information provided is available freely to the public online and in books you can find at any store. This section is not meant to replace a nutritionist or dietitian. In fact, I strongly recommend that you consult a dietitian and/or nutritionist during this month so they can give you more specific recommendations.*

The planning stage for diet is a little different (and easier in my opinion). There is an overabundance of diet information out there. What you want to do is create a well-balanced selection of foods for yourself. There are many books and thousands of research articles that talk about very specific, strict diets/meal plans. In theory, these will work very well and you are more than welcome to do this if you choose. I would like to caution you however, that diets that require rigid dedication to the plan with little room for enjoyment tend to have a ridiculously high failure rate long-term. Over the next few weeks, do research online, at the store, etc. Educate yourself on what is considered healthy, what vitamins you want in your diet, etc. (I will provide some more information in the diet chapter). I advise consulting a dietitian and/or nutritionist (a lot of times these are the same person).

## **"Should Haves" for Your Diet**

1. Eat whole grains and avoid white bread/white flour.
2. Eat colorful meals. Add color to your diet with fruits and veggies.
3. Variety over same old-same old. Change up your diet; eat different things so you do not get sick of foods.
4. It is ok to have dessert. Do not eat cheesecake every night, but once or twice a month; it is healthy (mentally/behaviorally) to do this. If you starve yourself of sweet things you enjoy, you will only crave them more. When you do finally break down, you'll over eat.

5. Eat different types of foods. Eat pasta, red meat, poultry, fruits, veggies, nuts, legumes, sweets, fatty foods, and foods high in protein. There are important nutrients in all foods. Eating a wide variety insures you get them all.

6. Portion sizes. This could not be more important. You can eat most things and be healthy if you consume the proper portion sizes. Take a small plate of food and eat that first. This will help trick your brain into eating less by thinking you are eating more. A general rule of thumb is that a portion size is about the size of your fist. So if you only want to have one serving of meat at dinner, do not eat half the cow. Eat slowly. Eating slowly will help give you the feeling of fullness while eating less food.

7. Healthy snacks. Where most people knock out a boatload of calories they do not need is with snacks and drinks. Try healthy snacks (yogurt, nuts, and fruits) rather than the greasy kind. Try drinking more water rather than fruit juice/soda.

8. Eat Organic. Yes, it is more expensive, but it is much healthier for you in the long run (less preservatives, etc).

9. Eat in. Eating out a lot increases your intake of sugar, salt, and the bad kinds of fat.

10. Do not overhaul your diet all at once. This leads to long-term failure. If you eat steak and eggs for breakfast every morning, do not switch to nuts and berries the next morning. The carnivore in you will not appreciate the immediate reversal. Make the switch very gradually over time.

11. Mediterranean foods. All of the new research is supporting Mediterranean foods (fish, oils, etc) for brain function and overall health.

What are healthy foods you already like?

1. _____
2. _____
3. _____

What are some healthy foods you'd be willing to try adding to your normal diet?

1. _____
2. _____
3. _____

How many servings do you eat in one sitting on average?
Meats _____
Fruits/veggies_____
Sweets _____

*Motivation*

Motivation is a tricky thing. What motivates people to do what they do is an extremely complicated issue because everyone is unique.

Finding that internal drive is truly the only thing that will work over the long term. There are all sorts of gimmicks to get you through the short-term, but at the end of the day, it is on you.

What motivates me?
1. _____
2. _____
3. _____
4. _____
5. _____

Month 1 is all done. Take some time and go through the checklist. Make sure you have everything done before moving on to month 2.


Month 1 Checklist

1. Have found time in my schedule to work out ☐

2. Have someone to workout with ☐

3. Have started trying new healthy foods ☐

4. Have equipment and/or gym membership ☐

5. Have set aside money that I will need to succeed ☐

6. Have various exercises I want to try ☐

7. Have a calendar/journal to write everything down in ☐

8. Have come up with some things that motivate me and some ways to try and motivate myself. ☐

Use this space to jot any notes/reminders down.

# Month 2: Motivation

*Goal: Set up a system that will motivate you. Do you need rewards? How often? Decide what type of motivation will work best in the short and long term.*

What type of motivation do you think you respond best to?

1. _____
2. _____
3. _____

I am going to do my best in this section to give you some strategies and suggestions. At the end of the day, this falls on you. There are countless theories and methods proposed on how to motivate people. I think it falls on the shoulders of the individual. What can you do to encourage yourself to change? **Do you want to change?** I've worked with thousands of people that have come up with all kinds of techniques and strategies. The only one that I have seen work for the long term is when people **want to change**.

*Scare Tactics*

Scare tactics have a certain appeal to them. Threats of cancer, early death, etc. have a certain resonance to them. The problem with threats is that everyone has heard them. We are threatened every day not to do this, or eat that. This is especially true for people who are already unhealthy. They have doctors, therapists, family members, friends, etc. telling them to change, "or else". Unfortunately we become numb to the threats.

On the way to get my drivers license, my dad made a detour and took me through the Intensive Care Unit of the hospital to meet a number of paralyzed and dismembered patients and just chat with them. They were all driving related accidents, as I am sure you have already guessed. I can assure you that I always buckle up, drive real slow, and will not drive after even a drop of alcohol has hit my tongue. It worked because I had never been in there before. I did not meet these poor injured people every day for 16 years. It is harder to use this same tactic with health related issues that occur over time. People always say, "I am not that bad" or "I will change before it ever gets that bad". Long story short, scaring doesn't work well with the general population and I would suggest not using that as your primary source of motivation. If people are not afraid of the warning labels printed on every pack of cigarettes threatening, cancer, death, harm to pregnancies, etc., then obviously scare tactics and warnings do very little to motivate people to change in the long run. To have a lasting effect, a true lifestyle change, you have to want to do it.

*Yummy Yummy Food*

A lot of people use food as a reward for exercising a lot and/or sticking with a strict diet. In theory, this is a great idea. In practice, it can hurt you more than help if you are not careful.

What foods do you enjoy eating on a regular basis?
1. _____
2. _____
3. _____
4. _____
5. _____

What foods are your "treats"?
1. _____
2. _____
3. _____
4. _____

If these foods are completely different, we are in good shape. This would mean that you are eating healthier on a daily basis and having your treats only occasionally. If you eat a treat once a week, or better yet, a month, you are doing well. If there is a food that is on both of these lists, we have a couple problems. It means you are more than likely eating too much junk food (as are most Americans). It can also mean that you are treating/rewarding yourself too often. Herein lies the primary problem with using food as a reward.  Most people will start by saying, "I can eat out and get a cheesecake once a month if I stick to my new lifestyle plan as a reward".  Once a month is fantastic and will do you no long-term harm.  In fact, letting yourself splurge occasionally provides motivation and offers a break from a new healthy diet.  It will feed your body's (or in most cases, your mind's) craving for fat and sweets.  The problem is that most people do not stick to this; once a month quickly becomes once every two weeks, once a week, and so on.  If you have the strength and will power, go for it.  If you know (and you know who you are) that this can only work for so long, do not even start using food as a reward.

*Entertainment*

What types of entertainment do you enjoy (think music, movies, etc.)?
1. _____
2. _____
3. _____
4. _____
5. _____

Buying yourself something at the end of each month is a common motivator.  I had a patient recently state when she reached 130° of knee flexion, that she was taking $100 to a casino.  She had a knee replacement and was struggling with motivating herself to do the work necessary at home to get better.  She set this reward up and quickly achieved her goal.  I had another patient with a similar surgery that traded in his truck for a tiny sports car that he had wanted all his life.  He quickly attained his goals allowing him to comfortably ride in his car.  Allowing yourself to spend a little money you normally would not is a good motivational tool (please make sure you have the budget available to do this!).

I rewarded myself with concert tickets.  Each month, for the first year I would purchase two concert tickets to local and popular bands.  This achieved two purposes.  First of all, I had serious motivation to stick with my goals because there was always another concert I wanted to go to.  Secondly, by buying the second ticket, I included friends and loved ones in my efforts.  If you do this enough, you start associating your exercise accomplishments with the great excitement and feelings from going to concerts (or whatever it is that motivates you!). Obviously, money is a consideration. Do not set this as your reward system if you are not going to follow through. It is not going to take long for you to interest in your goals without any kind of reward!

What are some activities you would want to go to?
1. _____
2. _____
3. _____
4. _____
5. _____

*Putting Your Feet Up*

Breaks can be used as a form of reward. I caution the use of these because they tend to be overused. The other reason this is not the best idea is that this lifestyle change is supposed to be fun. It should be something you want to do, so giving yourself a day off as a reward just seems counterproductive. If used appropriately, the break can be a good idea.

Making lifestyle changes are hard and sometimes it helps to have a day off. To avoid the usual pitfalls, try scheduling your breaks ahead of time on a calendar. Fight the urges to take extra breaks or add one here and there. If you are taking Sundays off, stick to it. An excellent thing to do is to have a journal or large calendar to record your activities on. If you did not do anything one day, mark it out with a big "X" to make it clear you did not do anything. It will serve as a great visual cue if you start seeing a lot of big red X's.

What can you do during your days off to make them productive?
1. _____
2. _____
3. _____
4. _____
5. _____

*Clothing*

Clothing is a popular reward system. It tends to be a more effective reward for women, but can be used for a lot of men. The idea is that at the end of the month, if you have achieved your goals and maintained your goals from the previous month, you buy yourself something. This can be a new pair of shoes, shirt, pants, a manicure, etc. It should be something you want or have wanted and will be excited to have. This is an effective way of improving your self-image, or how you view yourself. If you are working hard at changing your lifestyle and are starting to lose weight, gain muscle, feel better, getting new clothes can add to your newfound confidence and encourage you to continue improving.

A lot of people just want to reward themselves with things they want. This can be anything from a movie/video game to dinner out. Just like the clothing, it is effective. Just like the clothing, make sure you have it in the budget before you plan on treating yourself with "stuff" every time you meet a goal.

*Intrinsic Strategies*

The age of blogging and social networking sites has opened a new a relatively un-used opportunity (I have provided a blog to complement information in this book to further assist you→http://www.TheSmartLifeSeries.com/Smart-Life). Sometimes it feels good when other people know about your accomplishments and know what you are doing. One way to include everyone and let them know how you are doing is by creating a blog. At the end of each week you do an entry with pictures and stories from your past week, goals you have accomplished, helpful articles you have found etc. This way you can chart your path (and have people follow you). It has the added benefit of helping other people. They can see how and what you are doing and get motivated or be given some guidance on how to make changes of their own! Recording what you do and when you are doing it can show you just how much you are doing (like the calendar idea earlier). It is harder to kid yourself when everything is written out in front of you. If you like the idea of keeping notes on your progress, but not advertising it, getting a spiral bound notebook or journal can be a way to do that.

The absolute best kind of motivation is also the hardest for a lot of people to muster up enough of. Everyone wants to look better. But you need something at a slightly higher level than that (although looking better always helps). We need to feel good. We need to feel like we have accomplished something. Turn this into a challenge that you are up against. You want to win. You want to feel good at the end of the day everyday. You need internal motivation. You should feel good about your accomplishments. Make getting healthier a challenge that you succeed at daily.

Let's circle back to the *adherence* conversation because so much of that has to do specifically with motivation and the desire to change. I know we have already covered this topic, but it is central to the success of your lifestyle change and is worth reviewing. Remember that various research reports that approx. 50% of all people who start a program like this will drop out within 6 months. A lot of the dropouts are due to poor planning and a lot of it is that people just lose interest. I'm routinely told:
"I just wasn't seeing the results."
"I got bored."
"I never reached my goals."
All of these comments show a lack of motivation to continue, but why did this fail? What about all the work we've already done figuring out what motivates you? Some of it has to do with our perception of how things are going. You are motivated to change, but what if week after week you are not noticing what you think you should be noticing (drastic weight loss, huge muscles, etc).

1. **Make sure your first few workouts are relatively brief and manageable.** Some people don't like how exercise feels initially. Starting slow and gradually working your way up to longer and more intense workouts is a smart way to go. You can start out full of motivation and excited about change, but if you feel absolutely miserable, sooner or later even the most motivated person will lose interest.

What are some quick and painless exercises you can do to start?

1. _____
2. _____
3. _____
4. _____
5. _____

What new and healthy things can you start to incorporate into your meals that you will not hate every bite of?
1. _____
2. _____
3. _____
4. _____
5. _____

2. **Have attainable short and long-term goals.** For example: "I will exercise 30minutes, 4x this week." OR "I will walk 1 mile 5x this week." I will run my first 5K in 6 months. Set them up so you are achieving goals regularly. Have a weekly goal for diet and exercise. Make sure they are attainable. If your goal is to lose 20 lbs a week, you are setting yourself up for failure. What about:
- I will cook 3 healthy meals at home each week.
- I will exercise for 1 hr 3x this week.

What are 3 attainable short-term goals and 2 longer term goals?
a. _____
b. _____
c. _____
d. _____
e. _____

3. **On those days where you just don't want to move, make sure you do a little.** Do something like 10 squats, 10 biceps curls, and walk 1/4 mile. That way you are doing something and most times if you can get started, you will do the whole workout. Sometimes you'll just have to push through days. But hopefully those become fewer and further between.

4. **Variety.** This is the most important one for me. I get bored quickly. If I did the same exact routine every week for 6 months, I'd never exercise. Try new things. Add some flavor to your

routines.

**Sample Week:**

Monday: weight lifting for legs, bike for cardio. Cooked fish and quinoa.

Tuesday: Rock climbing gym for arms, walked for cardio.

Wednesday: Rest. Had a Mediterranean salad for dinner.

Thursday: weight lifting for arms, bike for cardio

Friday: did exercise machine circuit training at the gym

Saturday: swam at the pool. Grilled chicken and veggies.

Sunday: hiked. Read a good book and watched a movie with friends.

That is a lot of variety for one week, but you get the idea. People who do the exact same thing each week/month/year usually end up getting bored and quitting.


5. **Gym selfies are not cool.** BUT, getting people involved in this lifestyle change of yours IS cool. Hiring a personal trainer or starting with a physical therapist so you know what to do and how to do it safely is a great idea. These people tend to be your motivation in a bottle. They are always ready to go. Then get your spouse, kids, or friends involved. Find a gym buddy. Join an exercise class. I have a patient who is not a fan of exercising and I gave her this advice and her response was, "Why? Because misery loves company?" Maybe, but finding a gym buddy makes it more fun and makes you more accountable. A human being is meant to interact with others. Motivation levels sore when you exercise, cook, and enjoy life with other people.

Who can you involve in this healthy lifestyle?

1. _____
2. _____
3. _____
4. _____
5. _____


6. **Finally, monitor your progress.** Keeping a blog or posting things to social media is a great way to let other people monitor your progress. It will motivate you to show them how well you are doing.

This is a quick checklist for adherence. It is meant to give you a general idea of how likely you are to adhere to a healthy lifestyle and help you identify potential roadblocks. Each question can be answered: Very true, somewhat true, or not true. The more very trues you answer, the more likely you are to adhere to your program. If you notice a lot of Not Trues, it will be a good idea to go back to Month 1 and 2 to identify what you are missing before moving on.

1. I am very knowledgeable about physical activity and healthy eating.
2. I have a strong belief that physical activity, healthy eating, and finding intrinsic motivation is good for me.
3. I enjoy doing regular physical activity.
4. I enjoy eating healthy foods.
5. I know how to plan my own exercise routine.
6. I know how to plan and carry out a healthy diet.
7. I have a place nearby to exercise regularly.
8. I have a kitchen that is enjoyable to prepare meals in.
9. I have the equipment I need to exercise and cook regularly.
10. I have the support of family and friends to do regular physical activity and prepare healthy meals.
11. I have friends that enjoy the same type of physical activity I do.
12. I have friends that will cook with me.
13. I have a doctor/physical therapist/nutritionist to help me when needed.
14. I am ready to make this change.

Month 2 Checklist

1. I have an extrinsic award set up ☐

2. I have a plan for how often/how much for my rewards ☐

3. I am brainstorming good intrinsic rewards to use ☐

4. I have set realistic goals. ☐

5. I have people to share in this adventure. ☐

6. I have started trying new foods and exercises. ☐
7. I am likely to adhere to my program and I am ready to succeed.
☐

Take a minute to jot down any notes/reminders here.

This marks the end of the planning stage. My suggestion to you at this time is to make a master calendar. It should have each day laid out as best as you can. Because you have not had a month where you have had to make a major change to your diet or exercise, use this as a learning tool. Today, you can add hypothetical plans in. As you progress through the chapters you can add real things to your master calendar. For example:

| Monday | **Diet:** Breakfast (cereal, banana, water), Lunch (PB & J, yogurt and granola), Snacks (celery, grapes), Dinner (chicken, broccoli, wheat pasta, salad) **Exercise:** 2 mile jog before work, arm weights at lunch, stretching after work **Motivation:** Movie at the end of the week, blog entries **Planning:** Purchase exercise ball to improve core and leg workouts. |
|---|---|
| | YOUR TURN… |
| Tuesday | |
| Wednesday | |
| Thursday | |

| | |
|---|---|
| | |
| Friday | |
| Saturday | |
| Sunday | |

The above table is an example of what your plan will look like. We are going to take it step by small step and make sure that you succeed. I would suggest creating a spreadsheet/table on your computer or buying a large calendar or journal that you can fill in every week. It might seem a little tedious now, but it will pay off big in the end.

# Month 3: Diet

*Goal: Make the first meal of the day healthy and have healthy snacks during the day.*

We are entering the true "Action" stage of change. You are making a real, tangible change to your life in this month. It is time to "Put up or shut up." The goal above is your primary goal for this month. I am briefly going to talk about nutrition, then go into some options, and finally some suggestions on how to make this goal a reality and a permanent part of your life. Remember, you have the entire month to reach this goal. Start small and work up. Just a quick not before you get started. The diet section is a little long and I do not want you to get bogged down with specifics. I included a little extra only because diet is a big topic right now and I wanted to make sure you knew why you were making the changes I am suggesting. Read the "science stuff" but pay close attention to the lists and illustrations; I think they will help you. All of the actual suggestions being made are considered "lifestyle recommendations" and are not targeted at any specific medical condition. You will need to contact a nutritionist and/or dietitian for specifics.

What healthy foods do you like already?

1. _____
2. _____
3. _____
4. _____
5. _____

The first thing to do is learn about the foods you are eating. What are you looking for? What do you want to avoid? What do you want more of? What numbers are you looking for in your blood work? I recommend reading blogs, checking nutrition books out of the library, consulting your physician, and scheduling an appointment with a nutritionist/dietitian.

Cholesterol is something that everyone talks about, but few truly understand. Cholesterol is a component of the cells in our body found in animals (plants are cholesterol free!). We need some cholesterol for our bodies to function properly, but too much cnan cause trouble. Most cholesterol is synthesized by the liver (about 80%) with the rest coming from eating animal food sources.

Lipoproteins are the proteins that carry cholesterol in the blood. The two primary lipoproteins are HDL and LDL (discussed shortly). The bad thing about cholesterol is that the more cholesterol in the blood stream, the more atherosclerotic plaque that builds up, and the harder it is for blood to be pumped through the arteries and veins. This is where cholesterol (and other fatty material) builds up and can narrow and harden the blood vessel (a condition called atherosclerosis). This makes it harder for the body to pump blood through these vessels (raising your blood pressure). This becomes a very large problem in the case of heart disease, stroke, and various other cardiovascular diseases. You want your blood to flow freely through your arteries.

Cholesterol is not all bad—you need some. There is a reason your body makes it. Cholesterol is a precursor to bile acids (aid in dietary fat absorption), steroid hormones (made and released by endocrine glands in the body), released in the blood stream and travel to other parts of the body to affect change, part of the myelin sheaths of nerve cells (the insulation which allows normal conduction), and various other glands (adrenal, etc). Cholesterol also plays a significant role in the normal, crucial functioning of cells.

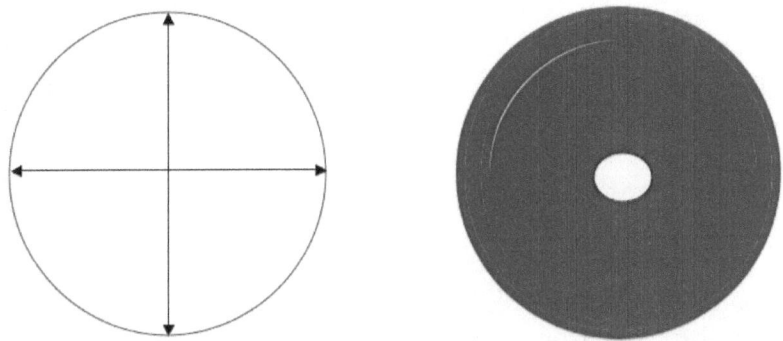

The above image is demonstrating atherosclerosis (when there is too much cholesterol). Just imagine if these vessels were providing blood and nutrients to your heart. The vessel on the left will allow significantly more blood to pass through than the one on the right. When you hear people talking about coronary arteries being occluded (blockages), the example on the right is what they are talking about. This significantly reduces the blood getting past this point in the vessel. This is important because blood carries good nutrients (oxygen, hormones, etc) towards areas of the body that need it and take the bad nutrients (carbon dioxide, lactic acid, etc) away for removal. Clogged vessels prevent this normal function from occurring.

HDL (good) and LDL (bad) are both lipoproteins responsible for carrying cholesterol. What they do with the cholesterol is their primary difference and the reason why one is "good" and the other is "bad." HDL's promote the removal of excess cholesterol from the cells out of the body. LDL's pick up cholesterol and drop it in the cells of blood vessels and muscles.

Hopefully the next question is, "How do I increase my HDL and lower my LDL?" There are many ways to increase your HDL's through lifestyle changes and diet. Quitting smoking is a good place to start. Cholesterol should be the least of your worries if you are smoking, but it certainly does not help your cholesterol. Losing weight is helpful. Depending on the source, 25-35% of daily calories should come from fat. Saturated fat should be less than 7% (this is where a lot of people struggle). Along with saturated fats, you are going to want to avoid trans fats. Monounsaturated and polyunsaturated fats (olive/peanut oils) can be a positive part of your diet. Other nuts and fish oils (omega-3) can improve the HDL/LDL ratio. Eat a lot of fiber. As bad as this may sound to some people, drinking alcohol in moderation is also suggested.

*After all of this, what are some foods you should start thinking about?*

Oatmeal, oat bran, high fiber foods, fish and omega-3 fatty acids (halibut, lake trout, salmon, etc), walnuts, almonds, non-salted peanuts, other nuts, olive oil, and foods with added plant sterols (yogurt drinks) are all high fiber foods that help remove cholesterol from the body.

> **Bottom Line:** Keep cholesterol intake to a minimum. Check your nutrition labels and make sure the foods you are eating are low in cholesterol. Eat things high in fiber to help lower your cholesterol. Speak with your physician and nutritionist/dietitian for more information.

*Triglycerides are something many doctors urge you to keep low. What are they? How do you lower them?*

Triglycerides are the primary type of lipid (fat) used for energy storage. When the body gets calories it does not need, they are converted to triglycerides and stored. In other words, if you eat too much (more than you need), it will get stored as fat. It is one of the mechanisms that make yo-yo dieting so undesirable and hard to stop. They can contribute to the hardening and narrowing of vessels as well. High triglycerides can go hand in hand with high LDL and low HDL (not the ratio you want!). Eating healthy and moderate levels of exercise (as for HDL/LDL) are the best ways to reduce your triglycerides.

*I just had blood work but don't know what I'm looking for...*

This is a combination of charts from the American College of Sports Medicine and the American Heart Association.

| Total Cholesterol | Level |
|---|---|
| Less than 200mg/dL | Desirable |
| 200-239 mg/dL | Borderline high |
| 240 mg/dL   + | High |
| **LDL** | **Level** |
| Less than 100 mg/dL | Optimal |
| 100-129 mg/dL | Near optimal |
| 130-159 mg/dL | Borderline high |
| 160-189 mg/dL | High |
| 190 mg/dL | Very high |
| **HDL** | **Level** |
| Less than 40 mg/dL | Low |
| 60 mg/dL   + | High (good) |
| **Triglycerides** | **Level** |
| Less than 150 mg/dL | Normal |
| 150-199 mg/dL | Borderline high |
| 200-499 mg/dL | High |
| 500 mg/dL + | Very high |

The bottom line is that you want your total fat intake to be relatively low (but still part of your diet) to reduce the risk of serious disease. Obesity and poor diet will soon overtake smoking as the #1 preventable death in this country. Eat healthy and start exercising.

Most people know fiber is extremely important part of everyone's diet. Where does it come from and how is it used is less commonly known. The good thing is, is that it is very simple!

Fiber is mostly indigestible and comes from plant sources. Insoluble fiber has a laxative function on the digestive process. Soluble fiber dissolves in water and beneficially effects cholesterol (lowers it!) and blood sugar levels (lowers it!). The positive effects on blood sugar levels make it easier to prevent/control diabetes. These effects are extremely important in people who are obese (leading form of malnutrition). These functions help control weight (lowering it). It also serves as fuel for your liver. Fiber helps keep stools soft and waste moving through the digestive tract. It is suggested that an average diet should contain 25-30 grams of fiber per day (some statistics suggest Americans consume less than ½ of that figure) and a dietitian/nutritionist will be able to give you the specific amount for optimal functioning of your body. These influences have also been linked to the reduction of gall stones and diverticulitis.

Fiber affects digestion from the moment it enters a person's mouth. It requires food to be chewed more (slows down eating process=feeling more full). It slows digestion/absorption (glucose/sugar enters bloodstream slower=less sugar spikes). The process in which it is dealt with in the colon helps nourish the colon's lining. Dan Buettner in "The Blue Zone Solution" noted that research has also found that high fiber diets are linked to decreased colon cancer risk.

*Food Sources high in Fiber*

All-natural cereals, whole-grain bread, fruits, veggies, nuts and seeds, bran (has highest fiber content), brown rice, legumes (beans, lentils, peas), oatmeal, berries, figs, and dietary fiber supplements all have high levels of fiber. Although supplements are helpful, they do not contain all of the important varieties of fiber gained from a well-balanced diet. For this reason, supplements should be taken in adjunct with a well-balanced diet and not in place of one. Surprisingly, fruit juice does not usually contain the fiber richness of their whole fruit origins.

*Versus Low Fiber*

Processed/white foods often have fiber removed. Any white bread/pizza foods are low in fiber.

*How to get more fiber*

It is recommended that high fiber diets be introduced slowly over time. Eating a wide variety of plant products will allow you to gain all of the major types of fiber. Avoiding refined/processed foods is important. Drinking plenty of water will assist in normal digestion. Eat real fruit instead of drinking fruit juices. Add fruit to your breakfast. Make sure the label includes whole grains/wheat/bran. Eat more beans. Try some international dishes.

**Interesting Fact:** Celery is high in insoluble fiber and actually has a negative calorie balance. This means that if you eat celery, you are actually losing calories because it takes more energy for the body to try and digest celery than the celery provides.

*Salt*

Salt is a major topic of discussion because of the crucial role it plays in our blood pressure (although some research is not as sure anymore) and its overabundance in most foods we eat. High blood pressure, or hypertension, is a major killer all over the world. It is highly prevalent in the United States. This is unfortunate, because in most cases it is highly preventable. At the very least it is manageable. The problem is that it does not have a lot of symptoms (the "silent killer"). Most people do not even know they have high blood pressure unless the doctor tells them so. Anything over 120/80 blood pressure is considered pre-hypertension. At this stage, you need to start making some changes to avoid any damage or progression of the disease. Things like diet and exercise are your first line of defense. 140/90 blood pressure is considered hypertension and you need to consult your doctor on the proper course of action.

Hypertension is a bad thing because it increases your risk of heart attack and stroke. There is new evidence suggesting it can damage your heart, kidneys, brain, and other organs in your body as well.

Salt is important to get into your diet for a normal electrolyte and acid-base balance in your blood. However, too much salt can lead to serious health problems. Salt has the distinction of being highly effective in raising your blood pressure. Added salt can lead to stiff arteries (atherosclerosis discussed earlier), kidney disease, osteoporosis, and left ventricular hypertrophy (where the heart muscle gets larger, in a bad way, to try and pump blood through stiff arteries), among others.

So what does this all mean to you? You must be careful when you are choosing foods to eat. Take-out food, food at restaurants, fast-food, frozen dishes/dinners, and Indian dishes are all extremely high in salt (Why do you think it tastes so good?) and should be limited as much as possible and eliminated when able. Your fruits, veggies, etc are all low in salt. Many foods are also coming out with low-salt or unsalted versions which helps. Make sure to check the nutrition label under "Sodium." The nutrition label will tell you approximately how much of your daily percentage of salt their product will pack in to you.

---

**Top 8 Common Salty Foods**
1. Deli meats
2. French fries
3. Bread
4. Chips, pretzels, popcorn
5. Spaghetti/pasta
6. Cheese
7. Canned soups
8. Pizza

**Daily dietary requirements are only approximately 2,300mg of salt. This is only a teaspoon!**

---

*Sugar*

Sugar (carbohydrates) has been the victim of a lot of finger pointing. A gazillion diet plans call for eliminating it completely in all forms (complex and simple carbohydrates). What these diet plans tend to neglect to tell you is that your body MUST HAVE sugar to live. Your brain's sole source of power (is your brain important?) is sugar. The reason for the finger pointing is not because of what sugar is, but what it can do in large amounts. If you eat it in moderation, you will be just fine! The problem is that most foods we eat have an inordinate amount of the stuff in them. Sodas, candy, donuts, refined foods, etc. have a months supply in every bite. In these quantities sugar can be extremely detrimental to your health. Type II diabetes is on the rise and costs the health care system something like ten-million-trillion-billion-gazillion dollars a year and is still rising. Obesity, high cholesterol, high sugar intake, and limited exercise are all significant risk factors for developing type II diabetes. Focusing your carbohydrate intake on complex carbohydrates (whole grains, wheat, multi-grain, bran, etc) is a much healthier alternative to simple/refined sugars and far less harmful to you even in larger quantities. Fruits and veggies contain good sugars as well. Again, inspect your nutrition label for carbohydrates/sugars. Try looking for low calorie/low sugar alternatives if you have to (ideally, without the artificial sweeteners either; which have been heavily linked to cancer).

Sugar is necessary in moderation and harmful in excess quantities. People always ask, "How much is too much?" A simple way to check is to look at the nutrition label and keep track of how many grams of sugar you are getting/day. About half of your calories in a day should be from carbohydrates (explained more later). The nutrition label will give you how much of your daily allowance you are taking in per serving. If the label says carbohydrates.........10%; this means when you eat a serving of this food you will have consumed 10% of your daily allowance for carbohydrates. It is also important to note that this is based on a 2,000 calorie day. Depending on who you are and your goals, you may be taking in more or less calories per day and will have to adjust accordingly. The common sense rule can be of service here too. An even simpler way to tell is if you eat white bread, drink soda every day, and enjoy ice cream and other sweets, you are getting too much.

| Foods with a lot of Sugar | |
| --- | --- |
| 1. Canned fruit | 5. Fruit juice/soda |
| 2. Canned sauces | 6. Muffins |
| 3. Pudding | 7. Cereal/cereal bars |
| 4. Cake | 8. Ice cream |
| **Daily dietary requirements are only approximately 20-30 grams!** | |

Before we go any further in our discussion about diet, I would like to address something. I was discussing a few of these topics with my grandmother and she looked at me like I had two heads. "I have made it this far and I am just fine," she said. She does have high cholesterol, hypertension, and emphysema, among other conditions. She believes they are fine because she has medications for them and she is still alive. She also tries to tell me about this friend or that friend that eat nothing but fast food and are "Healthy as a horse." This is a sentiment shared by many of my patients as well. The bottom line is just that some people are plain lucky. Sometimes their genes keep them healthy. However, the grand majority of people are not that lucky and not that genetically inclined. If you wait for it to get so bad that you need medication, damage has already been done and you are now in the business of damage control and rebuilding. Do not wait to act only once it is a problem. Be proactive!

The primary macronutrients are Carbohydrates, Protein, and Fat. Each gram of a specific nutrient contains a specific number of calories:

**1 gram of Carbohydrate has 4 calories**
**1 gram of Protein has 4 calories**
**1 gram of Fat has 9 calories**

Nutrition labels will give you grams of these nutrients. To get the total calories from each nutrient, use the chart above. If there are 10 grams of carbohydrates, multiply it by 4, and you get 40 calories from carbohydrates.

*The Real Deal with Carbohydrates*

Why should you eat carbohydrates? For the average person, about 45-65% of your total calories should come from carbohydrates, because the main source of fuel used by your body is glucose (carbohydrate/sugar). More specifically, the only source of safe fuel for the brain is carbohydrates. We have not talked much about the brain yet, but trust me, it's important. It is the primary source of fuel, because all tissues/cells can use it. They are important in waste removal and the health of the digestive tract. The primary fuel for any movement/running/exercise lasting less than 90 seconds is from carbohydrates. Think of what you do on a regular basis (at work, etc). Most things last less than 90 seconds, making carbohydrates extremely important to your normal functioning.

*Foods high in Carbohydrates*

Grain, bread, potatoes, cereal, milk, yogurt, fruit/veggies, nuts, beans. Remember from before that fiber is an insoluble carbohydrate (whole grains, fruits/veggies).

*Muscle and Cell Building Protein*

Why should you eat protein? About 10-35% of calories should come from protein. Protein is extremely important for growth and immune function. Although it is outside of the scope of the Smart Life Series, protein is also crucial for the production and normal functioning of enzymes and hormones. Protein can be utilized as a fuel source when needed. We will delve into this later as well, but protein is also important in muscle growth, lean muscle, and tissue repair. Every time we lift weights, microscopic tears are caused. These tears are filled/repaired by proteins and eventually lead to muscle hypertrophy (growth).

*Foods high in Protein*

Red meat, chicken, fish, cheese, milk, nuts, legumes (these foods contain the essential amino acids which are the building blocks of all proteins).

*Big Bad Fat*

Why should you eat fat? Isn't fat bad? About 20-35% of calories should come from fat. We want to limit fat in general and even more so for specific types (trans fats, saturated fats), but they are still important to eat. Unsaturated fats (olive oil, avocados, nuts, etc) are the kind you want to focus most of your intake on. Fat is important for normal growth and development. They form the lining of all cells called a lipid bilayer. They are a huge source of energy and can be stored (as most people know all too well). Vitamins A, D, E, and K are all fat-soluble vitamins. Because these vitamins can be stored for long periods of time, you can get away with eating them less often (less often does not mean the same as never).

---

**7 Common Foods Loaded with Fat**
1. Meat
2. Nuts (most nuts contain the good kind)
3. Dairy
4. Ice cream and other stack foods
5. Fast food
6. Butter, lard, cream
7. Deserts (donuts, cookies, pies, cakes, etc)

---

The next few pages are full of nutritional labels with explanations of the most important things on them! The first is just a blank one for you to familiarize yourself with the layout. Get a box/bag of your favorite food and compare. Find a label from a food you enjoy and write in the empty space below how much "good" and "bad" stuff there is in 1 serving.

# NUTRITION FACTS

Serving Size
Servings Per Container

Amount
Per Serving

**Calories**

Calories from Fat

% **Daily Value \***

| | | |
|---|---|---|
| **Total Fat** g | | |
| Saturated Fat g | | |
| Trans Fat g | | |
| Polyunsaturated Fat g | | |
| Monounsaturated Fat g | | |
| **Cholesterol** mg | | |
| **Sodium** mg | | |
| **Potassium** mg | | |
| **Total Carbohydrate** g | | |
| Dietary Fiber g | | |
| Soluble Fiber g | | |
| Insoluble Fiber g | | |
| Sugars g | | |
| **Protein** g | | |
| Vitamin ------ | | |

\* Percent daily values are based on a 2,000 calorie diet. Your daily values may be higher or lower depending on your calorie needs.

How many chips/etc equals a
single serving. This is important
because all of the numbers below
are based on a single serving. If
you eat 10 servings, you need to
multiply all the numbers below
by 10 to see how much you just
consumed!

This tells you the total
servings in an entire bag. If
you eat the entire bag, you
must multiply all the numbers
below by that total to get your
total consumption.

# NUTRITION FACTS

Serving Size
Servings Per Container

Amount
Per Serving

**Calories**

Calories from Fat

**% Daily Value \***

| **Total Fat** | g |
| Saturated Fat | g |
| Trans Fat | g |
| Polyunsaturated Fat | g |
| Monounsaturated Fat | g |
| **Cholesterol** | mg |
| **Sodium** | mg |
| **Potassium** | mg |
| **Total Carbohydrate** | g |
| Dietary Fiber | g |
| Soluble Fiber | g |
| Insoluble Fiber | g |
| Sugars | g |
| **Protein** | g |
| Vitamin | ------ |

\* Percent daily values are based on a 2,000 calorie diet. Your
daily values may be higher or lower depending on your calorie
needs.

If you are monitoring your calories, keep an eye on this number. It does not tell you anything about the real health content or nutrient density, just the total calories. This is commonly where everyone looks first. It is a good place to start, but read on.

This is a slightly more telling sign of the overall healthiness. You want to avoid foods for the most part where the calories from fat make up a high percentage of the total calories. On the whole, you want to limit your total fat intake.

# NUTRITION FACTS

Serving Size
Servings Per Container

Amount
Per Serving

**Calories**

Calories from Fat

% Daily Value *

| | |
|---|---|
| **Total Fat** | g |
| Saturated Fat | g |
| Trans Fat | g |
| Polyunsaturated Fat | g |
| Monounsaturated Fat | g |
| **Cholesterol** | mg |
| **Sodium** | mg |
| **Potassium** | mg |
| **Total Carbohydrate** | g |
| Dietary Fiber | g |
| Soluble Fiber | g |
| Insoluble Fiber | g |
| Sugars | g |
| **Protein** | g |
| Vitamin | ------ |

* Percent daily values are based on a 2,000 calorie diet. Your daily values may be higher or lower depending on your calorie needs.

## NUTRITION FACTS

Serving Size

Servings Per Container
___

Amount
Per Serving
___

**Calories**

    Calories from Fat
___

                                      **% Daily Value \***

**Total Fat**         g

    Saturated Fat     g

    Trans Fat     g

    Polyunsaturated Fat     g

    Monounsaturated Fat     g

**Cholesterol**     mg

**Sodium**     mg

**Potassium**     mg

**Total Carbohydrate**     g

    Dietary Fiber     g

    Soluble Fiber     g

    Insoluble Fiber     g

    Sugars     g

**Protein**     g

Vitamin     ------

\* Percent daily values are based on a 2,000 calorie diet. Your daily values may be higher or lower depending on your calorie needs.

Does 15g of something give you a good idea of what you are getting? Most people say no and this is where the DV% helps out. These percentages tell you how much one serving contributes to what you are supposed to get all day (based on a 2,000 calorie diet). So if it says 1 serving contains 10% of what you need all day and you eat 3 servings, that means you just consumed 30% of what you need for the whole day for that nutrient.

Your grand total in fat for the serving. This number is broken down below to give you a better idea of the types of fat.

The "Bad" fats. These fats lead to atherosclerosis and heart disease. You want these to be as non-existent from your diet as possible.

The "Good" fats. The research currently supports these types of fats as beneficial to you in small amounts. If these make up a high percentage of the total fat content, it is considered OK.

## NUTRITION FACTS

| | | % Daily Value * |
|---|---|---|
| Serving Size | | |
| Servings Per Container | | |
| Amount Per Serving | | |
| **Calories** | | |
| Calories from Fat | | |
| **Total Fat** | g | |
| Saturated Fat | g | |
| Trans Fat | g | |
| Polyunsaturated Fat | g | |
| Monounsaturated Fat | g | |
| **Cholesterol** | mg | |
| **Sodium** | mg | |
| **Potassium** | mg | |
| **Total Carbohydrate** | g | |
| Dietary Fiber | g | |
| Soluble Fiber | g | |
| Insoluble Fiber | g | |
| Sugars | g | |
| **Protein** | g | |
| Vitamin | ------ | |

* Percent daily values are based on a 2,000 calorie diet. Your daily values may be higher or lower depending on your calorie needs.

You need only very small amounts of cholesterol and salt (sodium) in your diet. Too much can lead to a multitude of heart and health problems. Keep these numbers as low as possible.

# NUTRITION FACTS

| | |
|---|---|
| Serving Size | |
| Servings Per Container | |

| Amount Per Serving | |
|---|---|
| **Calories** | |
| Calories from Fat | |

| | **% Daily Value \*** |
|---|---|
| **Total Fat** g | |
| Saturated Fat g | |
| Trans Fat g | |
| Polyunsaturated Fat g | |
| Monounsaturated Fat g | |
| **Cholesterol** mg | |
| **Sodium** mg | |
| **Potassium** mg | |
| **Total Carbohydrate** g | |
| Dietary Fiber g | |
| Soluble Fiber g | |
| Insoluble Fiber g | |
| Sugars g | |
| **Protein** g | |
| Vitamin ------ | |

\* Percent daily values are based on a 2,000 calorie diet. Your daily values may be higher or lower depending on your calorie needs.

## NUTRITION FACTS

Serving Size

Servings Per Container

Amount
Per Serving

**Calories**

    Calories from Fat

|  | % Daily Value * |
|---|---|
| **Total Fat**      g |  |
|    Saturated Fat     g |  |
|    Trans Fat     g |  |
|    Polyunsaturated Fat     g |  |
|    Monounsaturated Fat     g |  |
| **Cholesterol**     mg |  |
| **Sodium**     mg |  |
| **Potassium**     mg |  |
| **Total Carbohydrate**     g |  |
|    Dietary Fiber     g |  |
|    Soluble Fiber     g |  |
|    Insoluble Fiber     g |  |
|    Sugars     g |  |
| **Protein**     g |  |
| Vitamin     ------ |  |

\* Percent daily values are based on a 2,000 calorie diet. Your daily values may be higher or lower depending on your calorie needs.

Potassium is good for normal health and cellular functioning (including electrolyte balance).

# NUTRITION FACTS

Serving Size _____

Servings Per Container _____

Amount
Per Serving

**Calories** _____

    Calories from Fat _____

**% Daily Value \***

| | | |
|---|---|---|
| **Total Fat** | g | |
|    Saturated Fat | g | |
|    Trans Fat | g | |
|     Polyunsaturated Fat | g | |
|     Monounsaturated Fat | g | |
| **Cholesterol** | mg | |
| **Sodium** | mg | |
| **Potassium** | mg | |
| **Total Carbohydrate** | g | |
|    Dietary Fiber | g | |
|    Soluble Fiber | g | |
|    Insoluble Fiber | g | |
|    Sugars | g | |
| **Protein** | g | |
| Vitamin | ------ | |

\* Percent daily values are based on a 2,000 calorie diet. Your daily values may be higher or lower depending on your calorie needs.

---

Anywhere from 50-60% of your calories in a day should come from here. Just remember, that it is better if they come from complex/wheat sources.

Great for metabolism, weight loss, digestion, and general health. You want these numbers to be pretty high.

Every American gets way too much of this category. Keep this number as low as you can.

# NUTRITION FACTS

Serving Size

Servings Per Container

Amount

Per Serving

**Calories**

    Calories from Fat

|  | | % Daily Value * |
|---|---|---|
| **Total Fat** | g | |
|   Saturated Fat | g | |
|   Trans Fat | g | |
|   Polyunsaturated Fat | g | |
|   Monounsaturated Fat | g | |
| **Cholesterol** | mg | |
| **Sodium** | mg | |
| **Potassium** | mg | |
| **Total Carbohydrate** | g | |
|   Dietary Fiber | g | |
|   Soluble Fiber | g | |
|   Insoluble Fiber | g | |
|   Sugars | g | |
| **Protein** | g | |
| Vitamin | ------ | |

\* Percent daily values are based on a 2,000 calorie diet. Your daily values may be higher or lower depending on your calorie needs.

Protein is great for muscle growth and normal cell function.

This section varies greatly depending on how many/what kind of vitamins are present. You want higher numbers here.

75

*Organization & Suggestions*

Now that you have some background, let us organize things.

What are some foods you need to get more of?
1. _____
2. _____
3. _____
4. _____
5. _____

What are some foods you need to reduce in your diet?
1. _____
2. _____
3. _____
4. _____
5. _____

Now that we know what we are looking for and what we need to eliminate, let us get started. The goal of this month is to eat a healthy breakfast daily and eat healthier snacks.

What are you eating for breakfast on a regular basis?
1. _____
2. _____
3. _____
4. _____
5. _____

Look at this list and pick 2 things you can do without. Now replace them with a food you know you need more of.

**Say your breakfast includes**: Eggs, sausages, bacon, coffee, and hash browns. You decide you need the coffee to function, the eggs and hash browns to feel full, but you can do without the sausages and bacon. A banana and some grapes are a great way to improve your breakfast.

**Do you get fast food in the morning?  YES  NO**

What are some healthier options you can have?

1. _____
2. _____
3. _____
4. _____
5. _____

As with everything in this book, change should be gradual. Only replace a couple items in your normal breakfast initially. Replace them with healthy options you know you like (or at least do not hate). Over the course of the month slowly remove all of the unhealthy elements and replace them with healthy foods. If you need to move even slower, choose 3 days of the week to make these changes, and continue as before for the other 4. Work your way up to all 7 days, then all healthy snacks!

For those of you who think you have no time to make yourself breakfast and you "have" to go through a drive-thru somewhere, stop and think. How much time does it take to pour a glass of orange juice and eat a banana and granola bar? I just timed it, it took me 5 minutes at a relaxed pace with some reading thrown in. There are many good options for things you can take and eat when you get to work (depending on your job) including: bananas, granola bars, protein bars, oranges, a small cup of grapes, etc. Again, start doing these changes a couple times a week and work your way up to eliminating the drive-thru from your routine. Start preparing/planning your breakfast the night before. Fill your car mug with fruit juice or water, have a granola bar and banana sitting next to your car keys the night before.

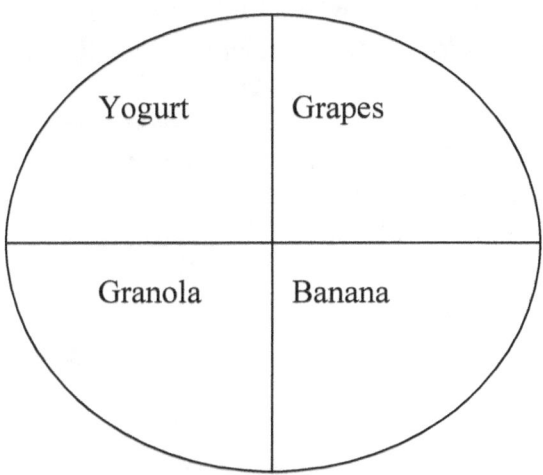

The diagram shows what an average breakfast plate will hopefully look like by the end of the month.  Obviously, these are not your only options, you are the boss!  Remember to eat a breakfast, even a small one.  If you have not had food since the night before, 9PM?, then your body is starting to wonder when will it get food again?  If you skip breakfast and wait for lunch, your body will enter starvation mode.  Your metabolism will be slower and by the time you eat, your body is prepared to put almost everything in storage (the nice way of saying fat) in case you try to starve it again.

The other part of our primary goal is to have healthier snacks throughout the day.  Many people enjoy chips, another quick run through the drive-thru, or a trip to the vending machine for something equally bad for your body.  More than anything, this takes a little planning.  You need something that is easy to carry and will fill you up in a pinch.  Personally, my solution has been trail mix.  I have a big bucket of it in the pantry with lightly salted pretzels, unsalted peanuts, whole grain cereal, raisins, and the occasional piece of dark chocolate.  You are going to want something easy to grab and something that won't spoil throughout the day.  Grapes, cucumbers, carrots, etc., usually need some way of keeping cool.  Bananas and apples are easy fruits to bring.  I personally need that full feeling sometimes, hence the peanuts and almonds.  Nuts in general are a good snack to keep you going.  Keep it simple.  The more complex and time consuming the snack gets, the lower the chances you will actually follow through with it.

The following table was created to give you a quick reference to common foods.  It gives you the most important information you need to know when selecting these foods.  I am hoping it will help you make healthier diet decisions, especially early on.  All the information on the table is given based on 1 serving (as per USDA).  Keep in mind that one serving of green beans might be a cup, but fried chicken might be 1 piece.  They are listed in alphabetical order.  Please also be aware that the way you prepare these foods will have an impact on all these statistics as well.

| Food | Total Calories | Fat Content (%DV) | Reason why you should eat it (or not). |
|---|---|---|---|
| Apples | 65 | 0 % | High fiber, vit C |
| Apricot | 74 | 1 % | High fiber, vit C/A, iron, potassium |
| Asparagus | 27 | 0% | High fiber, vit k, iron |
| Banana | 200 | 1% | High fiber, Vit C/B6, potassium |
| Blackberries | 62 | 1% | High vit C/K, fiber, manganese |
| Blueberries | 84 | 1% | High vit C/K, fiber, manganese |
| Bread (wheat) | 66 | 1% | High calcium, manganese, iron |
| Bread (white) | 165 | 1% | High sodium |
| Broccoli | 31 | 1% | High vit C/K/A, fiber, folate |
| Cantaloupe | 60 | 1% | High vit A/C, potassium |
| Carrots | 52 | 0% | High fiber, vit A/K |
| Celery | 18 | 0% | High fiber, vit A/K |
| Cheese (cheddar) | 532 | 67% | High calcium, sat fat, cholesterol, sodium |
| Chicken (grilled) | 231 | 8% | High in protein and cholesterol |
| Chicken (fried) | 809 | 75% | High in all types of fat |
| Chicken (nugget) | 83 | 9% | High in fat, cholesterol, sodium |
| Chickpeas | 269 | 7% | High fiber, iron |

| | | | |
|---|---|---|---|
| Coffee | 2 | 0% | Some riboflavin |
| Cucumber | 8 | 0% | High vit K |
| Egg (whole) | 211 | 22% | High cholesterol, protein |
| French fries | 539 | 44% | High in all types of fat, cholesterol |
| French Toast | 149 | 11% | High in fat, cholesterol, sodium |
| Grapes | 104 | 0% | High vit C/K |
| Green beans | 34 | 0% | High fiber, vit A/C/K, folate |
| Hamburger (plain) | 216 | 22% | High in fat, cholesterol, iron |
| Honey | 85 | 0% | High in sugar |
| Kiwi | 108 | 1% | High in fiber and vit C/K, potassium, folate |
| Lettuce (romaine) | 1 | 0% | High vit A |
| Mango | 107 | 1% | High fiber, vit A/K/B6 |
| Milk (whole) | 146 | 12% | High in sat fat, cholesterol, calcium, vit D |
| Mushrooms | 15 | 0% | High riboflavin and niacin |
| Nectarine | 63 | 1% | High fiber, vit A/C, niacin |
| Nuts/almonds | 167 | 23% | High magnesium, vit E, manganese |
| Oil (olive) | 248 | 43% | High mono/poly unsat fats, omega-fatty acids (good for you!) |
| Onions | 64 | 0% | High fiber, vit B6, folate, potassium, |

| | | | manganese |
|---|---|---|---|
| Oranges | 85 | 1% | High fiber, vit C |
| Pancakes | 175 | 11% | High cholesterol, sodium, carbs |
| Pears | 86 | 0% | High fiber, vit K |
| Pineapple | 74 | 0% | High thiamin, vit B6/C |
| Plums | 76 | 1% | High vit A/C |
| Potatoes (baked) | 278 | 1% | High carbs, iron, vit B6 |
| Potatoes (Mashed) | 174 | 2% | High vit C, fiber |
| Rice (brown) | 216 | 3% | High selenium and manganese |
| Salmon | 159 | 9% | High niacin, vit B6/12, phosphorus, protein |
| Seeds (flaxseed) | 150 | 18% | High in thiamin, magnesium, phosphorus, copper, manganese |
| Shrimp | 84 | 1% | High iron, selenium, phosphorus |
| Snap peas | 41 | 0% | High riboflavin, vit B6, pantothenic acid, fiber, folate |
| Spaghetti | 221 | 2% | High thiamin, folate, selenium |
| Spinach | 7 | 0% | High vit A/C/K, folate, manganese, iron |
| Squash | 18 | 0% | High protein, vit A/K, thiamin, niacin, copper |
| Strawberries | 49 | 1% | High vit C, |

| | | | |
|---|---|---|---|
| Strawberries | | | manganese, folate |
| Steak | 1,116 | 95% | High cholesterol, sat fat, protein |
| Sweet Potato | 180 | 0% | High vit A/C, fiber, iron |
| Tomatoes | 27 | 0% | High vit E/B6, thiamin, niacin, fiber |
| Quinoa | 103 | 3% | High folate, magnesium, phosphorus |

*How to incorporate all of this…*

You have all the background. You want to have a colorful diet full of essential oils, whole grains, and high fiber. But how do you get all of that? When do you have time to prepare all of this?

 Plan and prepare ahead!

It is the most simple, yet most effective advice I can offer you. This month's goal is to have a healthy breakfast each day and healthy snacks. Eventually, this strategy can be used for all meals. Pick a day of the week (Saturday or Sunday usually works best) as your preparation day. Get out some storage containers. I like the microwaveable and machine washable ones just for convenience.

Now chop, bake, cook, prepare your breakfast and snacks for the next five days, place it in containers, and in the fridge. Now you can wake up, grab the container for that morning, and everything is ready. This can save considerable time in the mornings. Sometimes it is even enough for people to fit in a 30-minute workout before work.

Yes. This can be time consuming on Sunday. BUT, it is amazing what it does for the rest of your week. It makes eating healthy so much more convenient.

The Basics.
1. Eat more whole fruits and veggies
2. Get color in your diet
3. Consume fermented foods
4. Eat unprocessed fats
5. Eat enough fiber from real food
6. Limit processed foods
7. Plan meals ahead of time
8. Make meals ahead of time
9. Whole grain not processed bread

Month 3 Checklist

1. I eat a healthy breakfast every day of the week. ☐
2. I leave out healthy snacks for the next day before I go to bed. ☐
3. I have healthy snacks each day. ☐
4. I consulted a dietitian and/or nutritionist ☐
5. I have healthy breakfast and snacks ready for the week. ☐

# Movement

Before we truly dive into the next 3 months (which all deal with exercise and movement), I would like to make something very clear. **Movement is GOOD**. So many people get caught up in the numbers (reps, sets, miles, grams, inches, etc) that they lose site of what is truly important—**Movement**. "So move. The state-of-the-art exercise science also points out, with increasing urgency, that inactivity is, for the human body, unnatural and unwise. Death rates rise when societies sit. Waistlines grow. Unhappiness spreads." –Gretchen Reynolds in "The First 20 Minutes." I will give you some numbers to follow only because I know people like/want the numbers to track progress. The bottom line is that you have to try and spend as much time moving as you can.

# Overload, FITT, and Everything in Between

How much is enough? What is safe? There is a scale from **Not Enough** to **Way Too Much**. It is different for everyone and something that you will find out as you begin your training.

I like to tell people "enough" is when you are pretty tired by the end of the workout, but not to the point where you are crawling out of the building. The next day, the muscles you used should be tired, but you shouldn't be in agony.

That is a pretty vague answer to a question people want specifics on but it is the easiest to understand. Now for more specifics...

**Overload** is necessary to achieve continued improvements in fitness. Overload means you must work above "normal" to achieve gains. This is true for the muscles of your legs, your heart, your lungs, everything.

Ex. Today running a mile makes you winded and you will get loads of health benefits from doing it. If you run that same 1 mile every day for 8 weeks, your body will get used to it and soon running 1 mile will not get you the same health benefits. It is still good for you, but your gains won't be as impressive. Maintaining a certain level of fitness is 100% OK. Do not think that you always have to overload your routines. But if you want to make gains, you will have to overload.

**Roadblock Warning**

If you have never exercised in your life, when you start, you will notice huge gains in all aspects of your health. The more you do it and the longer you do it, you'll notice the gains come slower. This discourages a lot of people. Just remember that attaining an elite level is harder than going from nothing to something. Let's say you are shooting free-throws in basketball. It is pretty easy to get form 0-20%. A few training sessions and tweaks to your form should do the trick. But getting from 90-92% is far more difficult and time consuming because of how technical you have to be at that level.

The benefits of overload only last as long as you overload. In other words, if you don't use it, you lose it. There is good evidence to support that you can maintain a certain level but eventually fitness will start to decrease. So it is important to always challenge yourself.

Challenging yourself does not mean punishing yourself every time you go to workout. It means slowly increasing what you're doing. Small and meaningful changes over time will more beneficially add to your healthy lifestyle than punishing yourself. It will also greatly reduce the risk of any adverse side effects from exercise.

The benefits you gain from exercise will be specific. If you only do biceps curls every day, don't expect your legs to get stronger. You will see gains in the areas you work at.

Exercise is like a medicine you take. If you have pain, you take a pain killer. The more you take, the less pain you feel. There is a sweet spot where the pain is gone and you are not harming yourself. Exercise is the exact same. A higher dose will yield bigger improvements. There is such a thing as too much exercise, although few people ever do that much.

*FITT*

Frequency: the amount of times you exercise. This can be looked at on a large scale, "I exercised 3 times this week" or a smaller scale, "I performed 30 reps of the squats."
Intensity: how hard you worked out. This can mean higher weights, speed, power, etc
Time: how much time you spent exercising
Type: what type of exercise you performed.

FITT is closely linked to your exercise dose. Increase any aspect of FITT and your dose will increase. This is why I recommend only changing one aspect each week in order to avoid any overtraining.
Ex. Frequency: 3x/wk
Intensity: 6/10 (self rating)
Time: 60 minutes each session
Type: cardio and strength
I recommend only changing one aspect. In this example I'd say keep everything else the same and bump it to 4x/wk. This rule applies for all types of exercise.

Time to exercise!

# Month 4: Cardio

*Goal: By the end of the month you will perform 30 minutes of cardiovascular exercise 3 out of 7 days in the week.*

Not many people enjoy cardiovascular exercise. Most people come up with a wide variety of excuses not to do it. Unfortunately, it is one of the single most important things you can do for every aspect of your health. It **literally** has the ability to prolong your life.

*Background on the Heart, Lungs, and Circulation*

I am going to attempt not to bore you, but I think that it is important to have some understanding of what is going on in your body.

To put it lightly, the heart is super-duper-extra-mega-important. It is responsible for taking blood in, sending it to the lungs, and then spreading it throughout the entire body to the very tips of every part of your body.

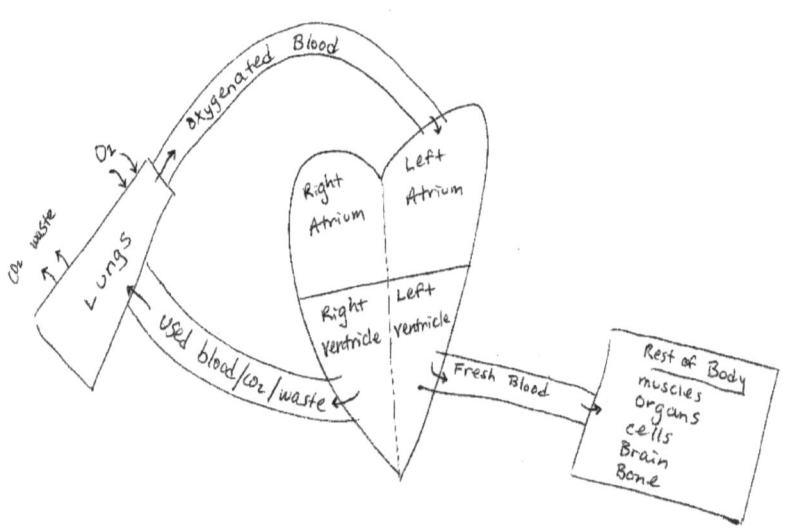

It takes in what I call "used blood", or blood that is depleted of oxygen and loaded up with waste (mainly carbon dioxide). There is a valve in the middle of the heart that sends all of this blood to the lungs where the carbon dioxide is breathed out and the red blood cells pick up the new oxygen you just breathed in. This blood is brought into the heart through a separate valve and this side of the heart then sends the blood out of the heart completely. This "fresh" blood travels through the arteries in your body and delivers all of the life-sustaining nutrients and oxygen to the working tissues in the body (bones, brain, muscle, etc).

When you exercise, the demand for blood and nutrients (like oxygen) goes up significantly. Even when you move from a seated position to a standing one there is an increased demand by the gluteal (butt) muscles that help you stand up. Your body needs to be able to respond. In some cases, you will need to work up to this point. Your heart currently has a limit of blood and oxygen it can circulate. By training, you can increase the capacity of your heart to work. You can actually reduce your heart rate and pump out more blood. How? Your heart gets stronger and is able to pump more blood every time. Remember that your brain likes getting blood and oxygen too. You want to have a cardiopulmonary system that is going to be very efficient at this task. This is hugely beneficial to your overall health and your quality of life.

The heart is the Hemi engine in your chest responsible for distributing the fuel. If you expect to move at all, your heart needs to pump all the fuel to the various parts of the engine. Each time it beats, the heart needs to get as much blood out to your working body as your body demands. If you can barely stand up and go to the bathroom or refrigerator without getting short of breath and/or tired, how much quality of life will you have? How will you be able to participate in hobbies, play with your children or grandchildren, or walk around the grocery store without a motor?

The more you perform cardiovascular exercises, the more efficient this system becomes and the healthier you become.

*Benefits*

What do you think are some benefits of cardio exercise?
1. _____
2. _____
3. _____
4. _____
5. _____


The following are a <u>small</u> sampling of important benefits:

Performing cardiovascular exercise on a regular basis will increase your metabolism. This means your body will burn more calories during a normal day (during the actual exercise and after you have stopped!). An increased metabolism will assist in weight loss.

Regular cardio will decrease your risk of heart disease, heart attack, coronary artery disease, stroke, etc. A lot of these diseases involve an artery getting clogged up by fatty plaques (atherosclerosis). Thousands of people every year require stents to open up "blocked arteries" so their heart gets the blood it needs. When the heart stops pumping blood, your body does not get the constant flow of nutrients it requires and bad things happen. Performing regular cardio will help open up and keep your arteries clear. Cardio trains the heart to pump more blood out with less effort. It allows a more constant, non-interrupted flow of nutrients. You could spend years talking about the heart, lung, and vascular benefits of cardio exercise, but I will spare you the time and just tell you it is **REALLY** important and does **AMAZING** things for your cardiopulmonary and cardiovascular system.

The benefits for the arteries around the heart, lungs, and brain extend to the whole body. Arteries all over the body become stronger and wider (by preventing fatty plaque build-up) to allow for the increased flow of blood to tissues in constant need. Cardio exercise significantly reduces the risk of atherosclerosis and has even been shown to help reverse it to some degree.

Cardiovascular exercise has been proven to improve self-management of diabetes. Cardio exercise increases the body's sensitivity to insulin and will decrease your blood sugar levels. If started early enough and performed routinely enough, people can stop taking their medications because the cardio is controlling their blood sugar levels (**consult your physician before making any changes to your medications!**).

Cardiovascular exercise has been shown to reduce stress levels and improve mood. Longer, sustained exercise bouts will have more substantial effects, but you will see improvements even with minimal activity. When you perform this type of physical activity your body will release endorphins (causing the runner's high) and make you feel good.

Cardiovascular exercise is important in increasing bone mineral density (stronger bones). The repetitive stress, especially on your legs, causes the bones to bulk up (increase strength and density) to withstand the impacts.

During cardiovascular exercise your blood pressure will rise based on how hard you are working out. The real benefit comes later. After exercising for a while, your blood pressure will actually go down at rest. This means that your heart will be beating against less resistance (which means better blood flow and less work for the heart). Once again, with the proper type and amount of cardio, people can actually get off of their expensive blood pressure medications because they have learned to control it with exercise (**please consult your physician before making any changes to your medication!**).

Part of the reason your blood pressure is decreased is that you lower the amount of fat in your body. This lowers cholesterol, triglycerides, and the risk of atherosclerosis (clogged arteries). At low to moderate levels of cardio activity, your body will burn primarily fat calories. Have a little padding around your midsection or thighs? Doing crunches every day will not do the trick. Doing crunches is great and you will build strong abdominal muscles. However, until the fat around your belly is gone, you will not see them!  You need to get rid of that fat and the way to do it is through prolonged cardiovascular exercise.

Believe it or not, exercising will actually increase your energy levels throughout the day.  A lot of people think it will wipe them out and avoid it because they do not want to be too tired the rest of the day.  Doing routine cardio will make your body stronger and more efficient.  This allows your body to spend less energy and effort doing routine tasks, leaving you loads of energy to spend.  Due to this extra energy, it is reported that your energy for other activities and experiences will improve—your sex life gets better!

Not to sound contradictory, but it also helps you get to sleep.  After a high-energy day with lots of activity, your body will want to recover.  It does not mean you will be tired all day.  It does mean that you will have a sounder sleep.  My brothers both have a torrid time getting any sleep at night.  They have found that if they are highly active all day and complete good workouts, then they fall asleep more easily.

As we get older, our joints break down.  Usually this is because we lose fluid as we get older.  The discs in our back and the fluids in our joints dry up.  There is no way to prevent it, but we can do a significant job delaying and slowing it down.  Routine cardio requires lots of fluid/smooth joint movements, which encourages the fluid to stay in the joints.  This leads to improved joint mobility and reduced joint pain.

The same constant and smooth motion that improves joint mobility also leads to improved flexibility.  When you use your muscles they warm up and relax.  This is why most research suggests doing a small warm-up instead of stretching before activity.  Think of your muscles like a rubber band.  If you stretch it cold, it is hard and runs the risk of damage.  If instead, you lightly move it around, it will warm up and loosen up and become very malleable and stretchy.  The same holds true for your muscles.

Cardiovascular exercise improves digestion.  This improved digestion leads to a reduced risk of colon cancer.  Teamed with a healthy, high fiber diet, cardio can significantly reduce your risk of developing colon (and other forms) cancer.

More and more research is now suggesting that cardio can reduce the risk of developing Parkinson's and Alzheimer's disease. Obviously cardio does not make you immune to these diseases, but it may reduce your risk. The research is not clear on any direct links; they are just noticing strong correlations. For people who already have these diseases, cardiovascular exercise is a crucial part of maintaining a quality of life. Cardio will improve your breathing ability and capacity to move around. It is imperative that you include cardiovascular exercise into your life even after being diagnosed. All of the above reasons still hold true, specifically (and more importantly) the pulmonary (breathing) and mobility examples.

The list below could be pages upon pages of various benefits ranging from the cellular to spiritual level. In case it hasn't sunk in…CARDIO IS IMPORTANT.

---

### What is Cardio good for again?
1. Increased metabolism
2. Decreased risk of heart disease, heart attack, stroke, etc
3. Increased pulmonary function (breathing)
4. Improved self-management of diabetes
5. Reduced stress levels
6. Increased bone mineral density (stronger bones)
7. Decreased blood pressure
8. Decreased cholesterol and triglycerides
9. Increased energy levels
10. Improved sleep
11. Improved joint function
12. Improved digestion

---

*Where is the time?*

If people have progressed smoothly through the first three months, this is generally where difficulties start to arise. Not many people like getting sweaty and tired. Some people feel they cannot set aside that much time in their day.

Fortunately, research has shown that exercise can be done in 10-minute increments as long as they add up to 30 minutes by the end of the day. 10 minutes of moderate activity, 3 times a day is your goal. You do not have to get sweaty and dirty or set aside a whole day just to fit in some cardiovascular exercise. "Moderate" activity can range from walking to football depending on your current fitness level (you determine the level). The goal is to raise your breathing rate and heart rate and keep it up for at least ten minutes at a time.

I have created the "Tired Rule" as a general guiding principal for you. If at the end of your cardio activity (the 30 minute total) you are physically tired, then you have done enough. If at the end of your cardio for the day, you feel like you can still run a marathon, you need to think about challenging yourself more from now on. As you get more used to this, try doing two sessions of fifteen minutes. By the end of the year, you should get a whole thirty minutes (or more) in during one session! Watch out; you might just enjoy it.

What parts of the day can you sneak in ten minutes for cardio?
1. _____
2. _____
3. _____
4. _____
5. _____

| **Tips for sneaking in ten minutes** |
| --- |
| 1. Set your alarm slightly ahead and get a quick work out in before your morning shower. |
| 2. Take ten minutes out of your lunch. |
| 3. Ten minutes right after you get home from work before you do anything else. |
| 4. If you shower in the evening, exercise ten minutes right before your shower. |

Your focus here should be to achieve a good well-rounded routine. Athletes are always looking to improve a very specific aspect of their game; you just want to improve everything a little bit. Your goal will be to improve your ability to pump blood and take in oxygen. This can mean walking, running, mountain climbing, and bike racing, whatever you want. Ideally, you will do a little bit of everything.

You have both aerobic and anaerobic pathways in your body. The aerobic pathway produces energy by using oxygen. The anaerobic pathway produces energy without oxygen. To sprint (or lift weights) or do bursts of energy less than a minute, we use the anaerobic pathway. A major limitation to this pathway is the available time our body can produce energy without oxygen. A side effect of this type of exercise is the build-up of lactic acid (the burn you feel). Once we have used up our anaerobic stores, we need to rely on other pathways or wait for the anaerobic stores to refill. This pathway is trainable. The more sprints and high intensity activities you do, the better your body becomes at producing energy, increasing stores, and removing lactic acid. It might seem pointless to train this for your everyday life, but it can come in handy in tight situations (running away from something, climbing stairs, etc). When you think about it, there are a lot of situations involving this pathway (lasting less than a minute): Standing up, going up and down stairs, getting in/out of a car, helping carry a heavy object, closing a door, etc.

The aerobic pathway is our main focus. We want to train our body to more efficiently take oxygen from the air, put it in the blood, and deliver it to the necessary tissue as quickly and easily as possible. To do this we need to perform longer sessions of exercise (greater than 1 minute, closer to 10 or more minutes is preferable).

How do we train these different pathways? We follow the specificity and SAID (specific adaptations to imposed demands) principles. All they say is that if you want to improve high intensity pathways, perform high intensity activities. If you want your cardiovascular system to be able to pump so much blood and oxygen over a 15 minute period, try performing activities for 15 minutes or more at a time to train that pathway. If all you do are short 10 yards sprints once a minute every 15 minutes, you will get minimal aerobic benefits because this is an anaerobic (high intensity exercise). You will make anaerobic gains. Train what you hope to improve.

How do you track your progress? How do you know you are improving? There are a couple ways. You can monitor your heart rate (check your pulse). As you become more cardiovascularly trained, your heart rate will decrease. Your heart rate should decrease at rest and go up less during exercise. If you run a mile on day 1 and your heart rate is 120, then on day 30 when you run a mile at the same pace on the same course, your heart rate should be lower (sign of aerobic improvement). Another easy way is the time test. If you can run a 100 yard sprint in 30 seconds the first day, but are running it in 25 seconds on day 30, yo have improved your anaerobic system (same holds true for the aerobic system and long runs). Distance is an easy way to track progress. How far can you sprint or jog before feeling tired? This distance should increase as you train. Finally, how easy was it? If running a mile used to wipe you out and now you are only mildly out of breath, you are improving.

Having some variety in your routine is important both mentally and physically. Mentally, you need a change every once in a while. If you get on the same bike for 30 minutes each day, sooner or later, it will be incredibly boring. If you are set and happy on only one activity (like the bike), vary your intensity. One workout sprint 10 times in the middle, on another maintain a moderate pace the whole time. Change it up. Physically it is good to place different demands on the body. You want to improve all aspects of your cardiovascular fitness. Include sprints some days, longer lighter sessions other days. This allows you to stress both the anaerobic and aerobic systems and improve them.

> **Variety Example**
> *Monday*: Bike 30 minutes at a moderate intensity
> *Tuesday*: Bike 15 min at light pace, 10 at intense pace, 5 min at moderate pace.
> *Wednesday*: Rowing machine for 20 minutes, elliptical for 10 min.
> *Thursday*: Rowing machine for 30 minutes total. Sprint the first 15 seconds of every minute.
> *Friday*: Bike 5 min, row 20 min, elliptical 5 min at high intensity

A lot of athletes use cross training as a way to stay in shape during an off-season without burning out. Eventually, your body needs a break from the same routine. If you run for 6 months straight and that is your only form of cardio, take a month or two off and try a different activity (swimming, rowing, hiking etc.).

How long should I go? Can I take a break? If you are going at a moderate pace, my suggestion would be to take as few breaks as possible to gain maximal cardiovascular benefit. However, if you need a quick breather and a drink, take it. Remember, doing 10 minute intervals 3 times during the day has the same benefit as one 30 minute session. The longer you can maintain an elevated heart rate, the more benefit you will get. If you are not up to that level and you can only do 3 minutes at a time, that is fine! Remember, everything is at your own pace.

*The Bottom Line*

A lot of people take the information from the past few pages and set up complex workouts and timetables. They want to challenge various physiological pathways and stress this or that system in different ways. Keep it simple. You are not training for the Olympics (if you are, you might want to invest in a different book). Get your cardio in any way you can and be done with it. The next few pages can act as your cardio journal for a while if you do not already have one. If you do already have one, maybe use these tables as week totals. It may be interesting to see how you are doing from week to week.

A lot of people suffer from aching joints, arthritis, etc. The table below will give you an idea of what type of activities to choose from. The no-impact column shows exercises that are kindest to your aching joints, all the way to high impact which are best done once you have been exercising a little while longer. If you do have aching joints, consider working out on softer surfaces when possible. If you want to walk, try finding grass to walk on rather than pavement. Be smart about this. If it hurts, look for a lower impact alternative.

| No-Impact | Low-Impact | Med-Impact | High-Impact |
|---|---|---|---|
| Bicycling | Walking | Jogging (slow) | Jogging (fast) |
| Rowing | Stair-Stepper | Jumping Rope | Running |
| Kayaking | NordicTrak | Tabata | Plyometrics |
| Swimming | Elliptical | | Soccer |
| Arm bike | | | Football |
| Chair aerobics | | | Basketball |
| Water aerobics | | | |
| **Date** | **Total Time** | **Activity** | **Feelings** |
| 3-30-11 | 45 (all AM) | Bike, Row | Negative |
| 4-2-11 | | | before, content |
| 4-4-11 | | | after |
| | | | |
| | | | |
| | | | |
| | | | |
| | | | |
| | | | |

|  |  |  |  |
|---|---|---|---|
|  |  |  |  |
|  |  |  |  |
|  |  |  |  |
|  |  |  |  |
|  |  |  |  |
|  |  |  |  |
|  |  |  |  |
|  |  |  |  |
|  |  |  |  |
|  |  |  |  |
|  |  |  |  |

| | | | |
|---|---|---|---|
| | | | |
| | | | |
| | | | |
| | | | |
| | | | |
| | | | |
| | | | |
| | | | |
| | | | |
| | | | |
| | | | |
| | | | |

|  |  |  |  |
|---|---|---|---|
|  |  |  |  |
|  |  |  |  |
|  |  |  |  |
|  |  |  |  |
|  |  |  |  |
|  |  |  |  |
|  |  |  |  |
|  |  |  |  |
|  |  |  |  |
|  |  |  |  |
|  |  |  |  |
|  |  |  |  |
|  |  |  |  |

| | | | |
|---|---|---|---|
| | | | |

*Obesity*

Obesity is an ever-growing problem in the world. People are trying all sorts of things to prevent it and/or control it. It has become so bad that over a third of children are overweight now and as many as two-thirds of adults are. Along with eating healthy and lifting weights, I feel that cardiovascular exercise is the most important factor. I understand that there are many factors that go into the obesity epidemic, but from what I have seen, cardiovascular exercise is the key. Cardiovascular exercise can help significantly lower body weight (do you see many overweight cross-country runners?). The lowering of body weight (and increased cardiovascular exercise) reduces the risk of heart problems and can control diabetes (Type II specifically) without medication (in addition to everything listed earlier in the chapter).

Even if pounds of body weight do not immediately come pouring off, it is still hugely beneficial. You will still see heart benefits, reduced chronic diseases, and improved mental well-being. It is also important to note here that lean muscle mass (your muscles) weigh more than fat. So you can actually reduce the amount of fat and not actually lose any weight. This is ok! A friend on my routine just commented on the fact that he is still stuck at 192 lbs, but he needs to wear a belt with his pants now or they fall down. His weight is the same (which had him discouraged), but he is thinning out already. He is just in the fourth month and he is already seeing noticeable progress!

Month 4 Checklist

1. I have the necessary equipment or gym membership to succeed in my goals ☐

2. I am currently performing at least 30 minutes of cardiovascular exercise throughout the day 3 out of 7 days in the week ☐

3. My schedule is arranged well so that I am able to fit in my cardio exercise easily without adding stress to my day ☐

4. I have activities that I enjoy doing daily ☐

# Month 5: Resistance

*Goal: By the end of the month you will perform 30 minutes of resistance exercise 3 out of 7 days in the week.*

**Roadblock Warning**

Soreness. If you have never exercised before or if you only rarely exercised lightly, you may never have felt post-exercise muscle soreness (or DOMS—Delayed Onset Muscle Soreness). This type of soreness lasts 24-48 hours after physical activity. This does not mean you are injured. This is **normal** after new and/or heavy physical activity, especially strength training. If it lasts longer than 2 days, get in to see your physical therapist to see if anything further is needed.

Resistance training and weight lifting are usually synonymous, but do not have to be. Resistance exercises just involve you moving your body, or part of your body, against some resistance—simple right? It can be as small as the force of gravity (which can be significant). Most people picture resistance training as going to a large gym and lifting enormous hunks of iron up over your head. In reality, it just involves you moving a body part against something that is above what is normally required of that body part.

## Background on Muscle and Nerves

Each muscle is actually a group of muscle fibers bundled together. When you want to lift something, make that muscle contract, your brain sends a signal down to the muscle and stimulates as much of the muscle as it needs to perform that task. If you are lifting only the weight of your arm, only a small percentage of your muscle will contract to get the job done. If you lift a really heavy weight, your body will recruit every last bit of the muscle and any muscles around it that might help, to lift that weight. This is an important concept for us. If one of your goals is to build muscle, then you will have to lift something heavy enough to make you tired. If you only lift light weights, your body does not have to try very hard to get the job done. Lifting light weights/high repetitions every day will not build up your strength nearly as much as lifting very heavy weights/low repetitions. You can actually train more nerves to be involved in the contraction of a muscle. If you are constantly lifting heavy weights and trying really hard to accomplish something, more nerves need to be recruited to make more fibers contract. By stimulating more nerve fibers to fire, you will notice significant gains in your muscle strength before you ever see your muscles grow. If you continue to lift heavier and heavier weights, you will see improvements in your muscle size as well. If your goal is endurance and not strength, the low weight/high repetition route will be best for you. The downside with this path is that you will not get nearly the same amount of benefits from strength and resistance training as you would from high weight/low repetition activities.

## Benefits

Resistance training leads to improved bone mineral density (stronger bones). Lifting weights puts an increased stress on your bones (specifically the involved ones). Your bones respond to this stress by making themselves stronger to avoid any injury (just as your muscles and cardiovascular system do). Increased bone strength prevents fractures, osteoporosis, etc. Especially as you get older, bone strength becomes crucial. A significant portion of elderly people who fracture their hip, die in the 1st year after the injury. A fracture in frail individuals is a long recovery process that some never succeed in. By around age 35 your body stops increasing bone density and you lose a little every year. For this reason we want to build up our bone stores as much as possible before that time. If you are older, do not think there is no point now. Doing regular resistance training greatly reduces the speed at which you lose bone density and some people argue you can bring that process almost to a halt (and maybe even reverse it). Stronger bones will allow you to have a greater quality of life as you get older.

The most obvious result of resistance training is that you get stronger. Strength is important as it allows you to interact in more ways with your environment safely. Being stronger allows you to do more around your own home and recreationally. It opens up all sorts of doors for you. You can do more for yourself without the aid of other people or machines. It gives you far more independence as you get older and reduces the risk of common injuries (falls, tears, etc).

Muscle mass has a faster metabolism than fat does. By increasing the amount of muscle mass you have, you can accelerate your metabolism (burn more calories) during and after exercise and lose weight and fat mass.

Improved mobility is huge. This is obviously more of an issue as you age, but holds true throughout the entire lifespan. Being stronger helps you improve balance. People are more comfortable on their feet with increased strength. You are able to stand up, lie down, and move around with far greater ease and far less effort with more strength. It makes the usual every day activities easy and not exhausting.

❧

One thing I would like to make clear before we go any further—there is no such thing as spot reduction. Spot reduction is the belief that you can do 200 crunches a day and lose weight around your stomach. This is just not true. You will build muscle in your stomach, but not lose weight right there. You may improve your metabolism and globally start to lose weight, just not specifically in that spot. For this reason, do not bother with those electric belts. If your abs are under a thick layer of fat, no amount of time with one of those belts on will give you the fake abs shown in the commercials. As your fat (all over your body) reduces, you will be able to tone certain areas (increase muscle). Put in the real work—diet, cardio, and resistance training.

*Where is the time?*

At this point, you have found 30 minutes, 3x/week to perform cardiovascular exercise. My suggestion would be to perform resistance training on the days you are not doing your cardio. Take the same times each day and just do resistance. If you are doing 20 minutes before work and 10 minutes of cardio immediately after on Monday/Wednesday/Friday, introduce 20 minutes before/10 after on Tuesday/Thursday/Saturday for resistance. This will help you get into a more regular daily routine of some kind of exercise or another. It will allow you to slowly carve parts of your day out for routine exercise. Another option would be to do your cardio immediately before work and your resistance 30 minutes immediately after on the same 3 days of the week. This will give you rest days in between. I would only caution that if you have not exercised much before, this may really make you tired and increase your risk of overuse injury initially. It also robs you of getting into a truly daily routine (which you will be doing eventually anyway!).

*The Whole Body*

This program was not developed for athletes; therefore, we do not have a small group of specific muscles we need to train. We want to train the whole body for overall wellness. The first mistake people make is wanting to train the "look at me" muscles (biceps, pecs, calves). These might be nice to look at and we will train them, but as far as your general health and reduction of injuries, we are going to want to train everything (front/back of legs, entire trunk, front/back of arms, neck).

Just like cardiovascular exercise, the goal is to get a total of 30 minutes in a day, but can be done in 10-minute increments. Everyone is concerned about how many sets/reps/weight. Generally, I tell patients 2 sets of 15 repetitions or 3 sets of 7-10. The truth is, you should do enough repetitions and weight to make you tired at the end. If you do 3,000 bicep curls and you do not feel in the least bit tired, you need to increase the weight significantly. For strength gains, do not do more than 15 repetitions in a set. You are starting to work more endurance than strength after that point. If it is really easy to do 15, increase your resistance. At the end of every set, the last repetition you do should be the last possible one you can do with proper form ("sets to exhaustion"). Proper form is key. If you start doing repetitions with terrible form you run the risk of injuring yourself (and you get less out of it anyway). If you have done a good workout, you will have mildly sore muscles the next day.

To improve muscle mass (if you want to see your muscles grow), the general thought is to increase total volume (weight x reps). It is important to note that you will see significant improvements in strength very soon without seeing a large increase in the size of your muscles. Neurologic changes occur first and account for the strength improvements initially. In other words, do 2-3 sets of 5-10 repetitions of a specific exercise. At the end of that, you should be seriously fatigued for whatever muscle you were using. I have found that, especially in beginners, the 2 sets of 15 rule works well as long as there is enough weight lifted to fatigue the muscles.

### Sample Week

1. *Monday*: 3 sets of 8 reps for the upper body.
2. *Tuesday*: 4 sets of 20 reps of core exercises. 2 sets of 8 reps for the lower body.
3. *Wednesday*: OFF
4. *Thursday*: 3 sets of 20 reps for the upper body. 3 sets of 20 reps of core exercises.
5. *Friday*: 3 sets of 15 for the lower body.
6. *Saturday*: 5 sets of 5 reps for the upper body.
7. *Sunday*: 5 sets of 5 reps for the lower body.

The next question is always how often? You should do it (this month) three times a week. You can do all three days in a row if you prefer. My only suggestion is to not exercise the same muscles two days in a row. Your muscles need time to heal and recover. Generally this means, exercise a muscle group every other day. Eventually, you will want to do resistance training for each muscle group 3x/week. Performing strength-training 2x/week is generally considered maintenance.

> **Ex.** *Upper body→Monday and Wednesday*
> *Lower body→Tuesday*

Remember the theory of specificity and the SAID principle. If you lift heavy weights 3 sets of 10 for your biceps every other day, your biceps will get stronger—your back will not. I know it sounds simple, but it is amazing how many people think by working out there biceps and pecs, that their back and ankles would greatly improve. Again, this is why we want to develop a program that trains the whole body. We want your back to get just as much attention as your calf muscles.

By the end of the year, you will be performing resistance training more days of the week and it will be better balanced. For now, I suggest doing the weakest muscles two times per week and your stronger muscles only once.

Resistance training also benefits from variety and cross training. If you do 3 sets of 10 biceps curls every other day with the same weight, your body gets very efficient at performing this act and will have to strain less and less to get it done, leaving you with less benefit from the exercise. Even something as simple as lowering the weight a little and doing 4 sets of 15 or raising the weight and doing 2 sets of 8 will present a different challenge for your body. If you do a lot of machine weights, try doing a few days or weeks here and there with the free weights.

Suspension bands are relatively new to the exercise world. I am going to take time here to talk about them because they are extremely space efficient with minimal cost ($50-120). They allow you to buy less equipment because you can do so much with them. They hang in any doorway. You can do hundreds of exercises for all body parts using a suspension band set. They use your body weight as resistance. There are upper/lower body exercises and trunk stability exercises. They can be used indoors or outside. www.youtube.com/TheSmartLifeSeries has pictures and videos of various suspension band exercises. Another alternative is the kettle bell. These can be purchased with an instructional DVD for anywhere from $25-$100. Most of the exercises with a kettle bell involve repeated motion of major muscle groups and multiple parts of the body working together.

Obviously cost becomes an issue at this point (if it has not already). Do you need your own personal gym? Not necessarily. My equipment at home consists of three dumbbells, a soft mat, resistance tubing, and suspension bands—a whopping $120 in total. If you are creative, this is very doable and manageable on a tight budget. Hopefully this part was already completed in month 1 and you do not have to worry about it here.

The following table has a list of many exercises. The exercises at the top of each list are my "Best Bang For Your Buck" exercises. If you only have time for a few exercises, these are your go to moves (please remember that this is not an all-inclusive list).

| Upper Body | Trunk | Lower Body |
|---|---|---|
| Bicep Curls | Bridges | Squats |
| Triceps Pushes | Posterior-pelvic tilt | Lunges |
| Shoulder Abduction | Crunches | Heel raises |
| Shoulder External | Planks | Step-ups |
| Rotation | Heel Taps | Side lying hip |
| Shoulder Internal | Crunches with twist | abduction |
| Rotation | Crunch Bikes | |
| Scapula Squeezes | | |
| Chest Press | | |
| Serratus Punches | | |

The table below will be your resistance-training journal for at least the next month.

| Mon | Tues | Wed | Thurs | Fri | Sat | Sun |
|---|---|---|---|---|---|---|
| Legs (15min AM) Legs (15 min PM) | | Arms (20min AM) Arms (10min PM) | | | Arms (20min AM) Arms (10min PM) | |
| | | | | | | |
| | | | | | | |
| | | | | | | |
| | | | | | | |
| | | | | | | |
| | | | | | | |
| | | | | | | |

| | | | | | |
|---|---|---|---|---|---|
| | | | | | |

Month 5 Checklist
1. I have all the necessary equipment or gym membership to

succeed ☐
2. I am performing resistance exercises for a total of 30 minutes 3

out of the 7 days in the week ☐
3. I have fit my resistance training comfortably into my existing

schedule ☐

# Month 6: Flexibility

*Goal: By the end of the month you will perform 15 minutes of stretching and flexibility 2 out of 7 days in the week.*

Flexibility tends to be a tough sell. Most people do not see immediate results which make it hard to convince people they need to do it. During normal daily activities, most people will not notice limited flexibility. If you do, generally it is a nervous system response to overstretching a tissue and not a limitation in the tissue itself. However, as you get older, flexibility becomes more and more important. As you get older, the elasticity of soft tissue in your body decreases (as water content decreases). It becomes harder and harder for people to perform simple tasks (getting in and out of bed, up and down stairs, in/out of a car). For this reason, it is important to start a flexibility regimen, even if it is only once or twice a week.

*What to Stretch*

I have found that the most important muscle group to stretch is the hamstrings. EVERYONE has tight hamstrings. I had a patient that came in complaining of low back pain for the past 4 months. His treatment was various stretches to improve hamstring flexibility—that's it! After 2 weeks, he was ready to move on with his life. The hamstrings attach around the back of the knee and up to your hips. If they are abnormally tight they can actually roll your hips down and backwards, putting extra strain on your back—a very common cause of low back pain. So if you stretch nothing else, stretch your hamstrings. The sciatic nerve also runs through the hamstrings and decreased flexibility of the nerve (neural tension) can actually result in what a lot of people mistake for hamstring tightness.

From my experience, you should also stretch your hips and trunk. Good flexibility in these muscles makes getting dressed, getting in/out of the car, etc. much easier as you get older. These are the most important, but a more complete routine will benefit you greatly.

As our world becomes more and more reliant on technology and computers, we see worse and worse posture.

Because of this, there is a great yoga pose that everyone should be doing to straighten out the spine after a long day of hunching over a computer. It is good for your low back and your neck. Lie flat on your back with your head and neck relaxed, hips and knees bent, and breathe deeply. Do for 5 minutes and do twice per day.

## How to Stretch

I have seen more variations of stretching than I have space to write about—everything from bouncing to just sitting there. Before any stretching you will want to perform a light warm-up just prior to stretching (something as simple as a 5 minute walk will be just fine!) to warm up the muscles. Think of your muscles as rubber bands. If you take a cold rubber band (your muscles before a work out) and start pulling on it, you run the risk of tearing it. On the other hand, if you lightly work with them and warm them up, when you pull, they stretch out much easier with less risk of snapping. The same holds true with our muscles. A more effective approach to prevent injuries is actually to perform a light warm-up (walking, biking, light exercise, etc.). To increase the length of your muscles (what I have been referring to as stretching), you want long hold times. My suggestion is 3 sets of 60-second holds (60 being the minimum). The old school of thought was that, the longer you hold a muscle in a stretch position, the greater the stimulus you apply to the muscle to add links and lengthen. In reality, there is no good research out there suggesting that you are actually lengthening any muscles. What you are actually doing with longer and gentler holds is inhibiting the nerve receptors that prevent your muscles from lengthening and relaxing. In other words, you make your nervous system relax and you can stretch more. If you have an extremely tight muscle, you should either do a light work out or put some heat on the muscles to help them relax before you start tugging on them.

Stretching and its use in athletic endeavors have been severely hampered by a number of persisting myths. Warning: Prepare to have your mind blown.

Myth 1: Stretching before exercise prevents injuries.
Reality: Remember your old high school coach making you stand around in a circle stretching for 30 minutes before a game? Well, he was wrong. I know you're thinking, "I see teams do that all the time even today." That's true, you do and all of those coaches are actually hurting the performance of their players. Evidence does not support stretching before a work out to prevent injury. In fact, static stretching (3 sets, 60-second holds) has been shown to

decrease the power a muscle can generate during sports and exercise immediately after stretching and can actually increase the incidence of injury. There are contradicting reasons for this, but the bottom line is that stretching before exercise is not going to prevent any injuries.

Myth 2: Stretching after exercise will decrease soreness later.
Reality: There is no evidence to support the idea that stretching decreases muscle soreness after a workout and is more than likely a waste of time if your goal is to limit pain. Stretching after is effective only in increasing overall flexibility as most nerve receptors are desensitized after the exercise and more accepting of the stretch you're putting on the muscle.

Myth 3: Stretching makes my muscles longer.
Reality: As we already stated, the muscle does not actually lengthen. The nerve receptors are desensitized and allow the muscle to lengthen.

After all that, why stretch? That is a great question, as I seem to be knocking down the merits of stretching. However, maintaining a certain tolerance for tissue stretch in the muscles and tendon is still a highly beneficial thing for daily life. You want to have the flexibility to bend over and tie your shoes. Bottom Line: keep stretching.

*How Often to Stretch*

The answer varies widely depending on what you read and whom you will talk to. What I tell all of my patients is—anytime you can, anytime you think about it. The following is my opinion based on what I have seen and read.

The answer will vary widely depending on your age and normal activity level. If you are younger (22 and younger), you probably do not have to worry much about stretching. A good, whole body routine once or twice a week will be sufficient (this is more than the majority of people do in most cases).

In the middle-aged group (22-45 year old), stretching twice a week should suffice. In this age group for the sedentary and/or leisure athlete, getting into a regular routine of stretching is good for maintaining normal flexibility.

In the older age group (45-older), I recommend at least some stretching every day. As you get older, your flexibility decreases. The reason why I suggest starting around 45 is that inflexibility creeps up on people and their activity becomes restricted before they know it. What I have noticed from most of my patients is that it sneaks up on you. I hear, "One day I was doing everything, and the next I could hardly look over my shoulder in the car" routinely. Flexibility is not something most people think about and it will catch up with you eventually. The older you get, the stiffer you get. At some point this will limit your ability to bend over and tie your shoes, get in and out of cars, move around in bed, etc. It becomes debilitating. Being proactive will help prevent the decline.

Month 6 Checklist

1. I am stretching at least 15 minutes 2 out of 7 days during the week ☐

Halfway There!

Congratulations. You are halfway through the program. Your life has changed drastically over the past 6-months (hopefully for the better). I hope you are starting to see positive changes in your health and are feeling better about exercise and being healthy. The next 6-months will be a challenge that I think you are ready for.

**Before moving on, let's assess what has happened.**

1. You successfully set yourself up for a positive change. By the end of the first month you had everything in place so that you could start your new life. □
2. You discovered what motivates you and organized a system of rewards and reinforcement in the second month. □
3. By the end of the third month you made the first meal of the day healthy and had healthy snacks during the day. □
4. By the end of the forth month you were performing 30 minutes of cardiovascular exercise 3 out of 7 days in the week. □
5. By the end of the fifth month you were performing 30 minutes of resistance exercise 3 out of 7 days in the week. □
6. By the end of the sixth month you were performing 15 minutes of stretching and flexibility 2 out of 7 days in the week. □

The table below shows what a normal week of yours should look like at this point.

| Mon | Tues | Wed | Thurs | Fri | Sat | Sun |
|---|---|---|---|---|---|---|
| Ate Healthy | Ate Healthy | Ate Healthy | Ate Healthy | Ate Healthy | Ate Healthy | Ate Healthy |
| | Cardio-30min | | Cardio-30min | | Cardio-30min | |
| Weight training 30min | | Weight training 30min | | Weight training 30min | | Motiva-tion: bought DVD ($8) |
| | | Stretch-ed 15min | | | | Stretch-ed 15min |

## Half-Way Point

Age: _____          Height: _____          BMI: _____

Weight: _____          HR: _____          Body Fat %: _____

Blood Pressure: _____

Waist Size: _____          Are You Healthy? _____

What goals have you successfully met?
1. _____
2. _____
3. _____
4. _____
5. _____
6. _____
7. _____
8. _____
9. _____
10. _____

Are there any goals you would like to add?
1. _____
2. _____
3. _____
4. _____
5. _____

# Month 7: Planning/Maintenance

*Goal: Assess everything you have accomplished. Look for things that tripped you up or need to be changed/improved. Establish an updated plan of action.*

If you have successfully made it this far in the program, congratulations! Most people are unable to continue with a new lifestyle change this long. You should be very proud of your accomplishments and ready for the new challenges.

Now that you have completed the first round of challenges and goals, it is time to assess what has worked for you and what has not (please continue with your program during this month, this is not a time to drop everything!).

 If you have not already done so, get a journal/calendar/blog/ computer program/or notebook of some kind to keep track of all your progress!

Here are just a few questions I came up with. They are regarding a number of problems friends, patients, and I have come across.

1. Is the gym too expensive? Is there a way to quit without being fined? Does the gym help motivate you to exercise still? Do you think you'd be better off getting your own equipment? Would working alone be easier for you?
2. Is your rewards system working? Are you looking forward to your rewards? Are you ready to make them less tangible (intrinsic)? If they are intrinsic, do you need the occasional tangible reward?
3. Are you enjoying the foods you are eating? Are they fulfilling your hunger cravings? Have you tried different recipes? Are you tired of your current diet? How often do you "cheat" on your current diet?
4. Are you enjoying your cardiovascular routine? Is it time to try something different? What are your options?
5. Are you enjoying your resistance training routine? Is it time to try something different? What are your options?

6. Are you enjoying your flexibility routine?  Is it time to try something different?

7.  Is it time for new sneakers/workout shoes (change running shoes about every 300 miles)?  Is it time for new workout clothes?

8.  Do you need a new play list to workout to?  Have you tried working out with audiobooks to help pass the time?  Do you prefer peace and quiet?

**Roadblock Warning**
People's passion and motivation tends to fizzle out during this month.  Figure out what you like to do and why you are doing it.  Don't forget about variety.

Now that you have looked at the past few months and have asked the necessary questions, it is time for you to fix things.  In the coming months you are going to have to increase your time invested in this lifestyle change.  Make sure that everything is arranged so that you can smoothly continue transitioning into your lifestyle transformation.  Just like the first planning month, this planning month can become planning "months."  Just remember that all of the goals you have met so far need to be carried through.  For example:  If this Month 7 takes you 2 months, throughout the 2 months you still need to eat a healthy breakfast and snacks each day, cardio and strengthening for 30 minutes 3x/week, and flexibility for 15 minutes 2x/week.  Do not let the planning stage mean, "break."

What do you see are some potential roadblocks to continuing this healthy lifestyle you have created?

Examples from my experiences:
1.  Working out at home is getting boring.
2.  Joined a gym with a ton of equipment.  Obviously an added expense, but well worth it.

Use this space to brainstorm some solutions. Remember, there will always be roadblocks; you need to find a way to push them aside and move forward. You will be happy you did.

What are some things you noticed about the first 6 months? Have you lost weight? Do you have a more positive outlook on life? Are you uncomfortable, hungry, etc? Write out some pros and cons below. If you have cons, write out how you can fix them. Examples from my experiences:

1.  I feel more awake when I get up in the morning, especially after my morning jog.
2.  I feel like I am focusing too much on food and that seems to make me hungry→my solution was to have a bigger breakfast. I went from juice, a banana, and a granola bar to yogurt with fruit and granola, water, and some almonds. It was a situation where I wasn't eating enough and my body was telling me to get more food. I did not want to overeat, so I added healthy foods. That way my calorie count did not go up too much, but I felt full after breakfast and had quality food to get me there.

## Month 7 Checklist

1. I have corrected any problems and am prepared to move on with my lifestyle change ☐

The following blank space is to give you space to jot some notes to yourself (things to do, preparations needed, phone numbers, etc).

Use this space for extra notes, phone numbers, goals, etc.

# Month 8: Motivation

*Goal: Start taking tangible rewards away. You do not want to need them! By the end of the month, you will be intrinsically rewarding yourself.*

Finding something to motivate you is usually easier than this next step—taking it away. Just like a new puppy you are rewarding every time they use the bathroom outside and not on your bed, eventually you want to do these things without needing a reward. This new lifestyle needs to become part of your routine, not a chore. This is a very tricky part for most people. If you do not have something tangible to motivate you, why do it? It is another reason that internal gain is a great motivator, because you will always have that. My best friend loves the feeling he gets after a workout and actually looks forward to them daily. At the time I am writing this, I have been working out and eating healthy most days for the past 3 years. My drive at this point is purely internal. I know how important it is and I want to prolong my healthy years and quality of life for the rest of my life. Easier said than done. How do you do this, especially if your motivator is a "thing"?

The first step is to cut back, not cut out. If you are rewarding yourself every week, make it every other week. The weeks you are not rewarding yourself with something, sit down on Sunday and make a list of reasons why you are making this change. It will serve as its own internal motivation.

Week 1:
Ex. So I can participate more with my children in sports.
Ex 2. Because I take less medication now.

1. _____
2. _____
3. _____
4. _____
5. _____

Week 2:
1. _____
2. _____
3. _____
4. _____
5. _____

Are you proud of what you have accomplished and how it is helping you become a better, healthier person?  You are doing something that most of the world cannot!  You are changing for the better.  2/3 of the US population is overweight.  1/3 of the US population is obese.  1/3 of children are overweight (rising FAST).  All of these numbers are rising. YOU are doing something positive to change these statistics.  You are doing something to improve your quality of life.

Each month, remove one "thing" reward and replace it with another list.  This is a real list from a patient of mine.  This is a sample of her Chapter 8.

Week 1: Went to a local concert.

Week 2:
1. __Improving my blood pressure _____
2. __Decreasing stress levels _____
3. __I am now able to go on walks in the neighborhood with my granddaughter. _____
4. ___I can garden all weekend without my knees hurting _____
5. ___Losing weight, slowly but surely _____

Week 3: Went to ice cream parlor


Week 4:
1. __Feeling better about myself _____
2. __Lowered my cholesterol _____
3. ___Fitting into smaller clothes _____
4. ___Spending more time in the lake with my grandkids _____
5. ___Rode a bike for the 1st time in 2 years _____

The next month she had recorded 3 lists and 1 reward and so on. I realize it is easier said than done, but it can be done. Your turn!

Week 1: _____

Week 2:
1. _____
2. _____
3. _____
4. _____
5. _____

Week 3: _____

Week 4:
1. _____
2. _____
3. _____
4. _____
5. _____

Week 5: _____

Week 6:
1. _____
2. _____
3. _____
4. _____
5. _____


Week 7:
1. _____
2. _____
3. _____
4. _____
5. _____

Week 8:

1. _____
2. _____
3. _____
4. _____
5. _____

Week 9:
1. _____
2. _____
3. _____
4. _____
5. _____

Week 10:
1. _____
2. _____
3. _____
4. _____
5. _____

Week 11:
1. _____
2. _____
3. _____
4. _____
5. _____

Week 12:
1. _____
2. _____
3. _____
4. _____
5. _____

I know you might be thinking that there are a lot of lists and you will not be able to come up with that many different things to internally motivate you. I think it will be easier than you think. Remember, it does not have to be different things every week. If losing cholesterol is still driving you, write it down! A suggestion with the cholesterol (and weight, blood levels, etc.), make it a challenge. Obviously you want to get the numbers into safe ranges, but set a realistic number for yourself and aim for it the next time you get blood drawn. I have even had patients (husband and wife) competing to see who can lower their cholesterol by the greatest amount safely.

*Ideas to Try*

Some people have had luck making commitment contracts. Again, I'm hoping you don't need something like this, but it is effective for a lot of people. A commitment contract is where you sign your own contract saying something like, "Every week I don't meet my goal of 30 minutes of cardio 3x per week, I will hand the next person I see a $20 bill as a penalty."

Write down how you feel after completing a good workout. Research shows that most people have positive feelings and feelings of accomplishment after a workout. Writing these feelings down reminds you prior to a workout you don't feel like doing how good you will feel soon.

Read a fitness magazine. There are many theories as to why this works, but the bottom line is that people who read fitness magazines want to exercise more.

Follow healthy living blogs and success stories. Reading about how other people are making positive changes will make you more motivated to make the same changes.

If you are ever feeling really stressed, head to the gym and take it out on the weights. Exercise has an amazing ability to decrease stress hormone levels in your body. You will feel better.

Post your success somewhere. By letting the world know how you are doing, you are adding a level of accountability to your routine. You don't want to let down all your adoring fans!

Month 8 Checklist

1. I am only rewarding myself intrinsically ☐

# Month 9: Diet

*Goal: Have a healthy lunch and dinner 6 out of 7 days in the week.*

The last time we visited your diet, the goal was to have a healthy breakfast and snacks. This time we are just upping the ante to include lunch and dinner. This is tough and will take some working in to. At this point you are already eating a healthy breakfast and snacks 7 days of the week. Lunch and dinner are a little harder. Hopefully by now, you are starting to venture into the world of healthier foods and are developing a taste for some new things.

If you haven't already, consult a nutritionist/dietitian.

Like all the other steps, start small. If you are not eating a single healthy lunch and/or dinner any night of the week, start by eating 2 healthy lunches and 2 healthy dinners each week. They can be on the same or different days. Like the exercise, I would suggest spreading them out so you are doing multiple meals (breakfast + lunch/dinner) each day rather than many healthy meals only a couple days of the week. Start paying even more attention to nutrition labels. Look for things high in fiber and vitamins and low in cholesterol and calories.

Sandwiches are easy lunches that you can make very healthy. Just remember that deli meats are loaded with salt! Bring a couple healthy sides to make sure you are full at the end of the meal (granola/blueberries and yogurt is my personal favorite).

Dinner is the real catch. By the time you get home, exercise, relax, deal with everything else going on in your life, the idea of cooking yourself a healthy dinner has long since left your head. What do you do? Fortunately, there are dozens of cookbooks with recipes that can be made healthily and in a small time frame. These are phenomenal and you should really look into a couple. Most will also include a nutrition chart which helps immensely.

One of the best tips I can offer you is to plan ahead. This applies for all meals and snacks, but especially dinner. An easy thing I like to do is cook too much dinner and have leftovers for a day or two for lunch. Another option is to grill/cook/etc a few breasts of chicken (or other meats) and then freeze them. For a few nights afterwards you will easily be able to pull out your frozen (already cooked) chicken, the frozen bag of veggies (frozen veggies have been shown to have more vitamins and nutrients than fresh fruits/veggies that can be lost trying to preserve them for supermarket shelves), and a healthy, complete dinner can be ready in mere seconds. If you see the "pre-prepared" meals in the supermarket—BEWARE. These tend to be packed with more salt and fat than you could ever imagine. Cook and freeze it yourself!

Lunch can be done similarly. Pack it the night before (right before bed) so you can just grab it as you walk out the door in the morning. Then you do not have to get up any earlier to pack your lunch in the morning (same is true for snacks).

If one of your goals is to get more fruits and veggies in a day, create supplies. Most fruits and veggies take a little prep (cleaning, cutting, etc). If you are planning on having cucumbers and carrots as a snack tomorrow, clean and cut a couple days worth tonight.

For all of these meals and snacks, you need to find some storage containers. I put my meals and snacks in a couple of these every night. This is a good way to watch your portion control and a good way to watch your progress (made 5 containers every day in the start, now its only 3), or lack there of. This only makes it easier for you. If you spend a few minutes extra Sunday night preparing all of these ready to eat meals for the week, things go a lot more smoothly and you feel like you are wasting less time during the week worrying about food. If you are trying to save money, this is much cheaper than eating out, even at cheaper restaurants.

Another option is a professional chef. Most people think that they cannot afford that, but you can. There are chefs that cook a weeks worth of food and drops it off at the beginning of the week. This reduces overall cost while increasing convenience for you. You

can get home-cooked, organic, and delicious dinners for $8.
That's not a bad deal.

The last thing I'll say is—do not prepare hungry. If you are sitting
in front of your fridge at 9:30PM Sunday night trying to think of
what to make for the weeks meals and you are starving, you will
prepare way too much. You will over-pack for the week. Just like
people say, do not go to the supermarket hungry, do not prepare
your meals hungry. You will over-pack and over-eat.

*A Few Sample Days*

| Day 1 | Breakfast: cereal, banana, water<br>Lunch: PB & J, yogurt with granola, orange juice<br>Dinner: grilled chicken, broccoli, corn, glass of wine<br>Snacks: grapes, carrots, cucumbers, wheat crackers |
|-------|---|
| Day 2 | Breakfast: toast, grapefruit, water<br>Lunch: grilled chicken salad, wheat crackers<br>Dinner: grilled fish with lemon, mashed potatoes, side salad, water<br>Snacks: yogurt, tomato and basil |
| Day 3 | Breakfast: scrambled eggs, toast, orange, coffee<br>Lunch: grilled chicken sandwich, side salad<br>Dinner: pasta salad, apple, water<br>Snacks: carrots, watermelon |
| Day 4 | Breakfast: cereal with banana, apple, water<br>Lunch: Ham and cheese sandwich, salad, juice<br>Dinner: Tomato with mozzarella and basil, fruit salad<br>Snacks: granola bar, yogurt, orange, celery |

*Research Recap*

Because most of this month is really just an extension of the
previous diet month (Month 3), I thought it would be interesting to
give you a recap of some nutrition/diet research. It might be worth
applying some of these principles to change things up.

The Journal of Marketing found that people are more likely to overeat small treats in clear packages vs. opaque ones. Out of sight=out of mouth?

The Journal of Public Health Nutrition suggests following the 10:1 ratio rule (10 grams of carbs to 1 gram of fiber). Foods that met that ratio had less sugar, salt, and bad fats than those that failed to meet the 10:1 ratio.

In the journal Flavour, they found that the less of a distinctive smell/taste a food has, the more you will eat of it. Just think of crummy fast food joints. Have you ever wondered why everything smells/tastes about the same? It is absolutely a sales tactic. So get lots of flavors in your dishes. This particular article recommends adding herbs instead of salt to significantly cut down on your salt intake.

A recent study offered alternatives to salt, which included: ginger, black pepper, cinnamon, cayenne, and mustard seed.

This one honestly made me get multiple references before believing it, but I have managed to find it in multiple respectable articles so here it is. If you are going to eat pasta, eat it cold. The Journal of Nutrition and Metabolism found that the drop in temperature altered the nature of the pasta making it a more resistant starch meaning that your body has to work harder to digest it=burns more calories.

A study in the journal of Psychological Reports found that people eating in a relaxed environment with dim lights ate an average of 175 less calories than those in bright high-energy environments.

Always choose the whole fruit over the juice. The Harvard School of Public Health found that people who consumed fruit juice daily increased the risk of developing Type 2 Diabetes by up to 20% whereas people consuming the recommended amount of daily whole fruits reduced their risk of diabetes by 20%.

A study in the Journal of Diabetes Pro found that people who drank 2 or more diet sodas a day had larger waistlines than those that didn't.

Eat an appetizer before your meal to cut calories by up to 20%. Something as simple as an apple pre-meal can do the trick (Journal of American Medical Assoc.).

Cornell University conducted a study and found that people that paid with cash were more aware of their food choices and chose healthier foods over those who paid with credit card.

According to the Journal of Clinical Endocrinology and Metabolism, drinking about 17 ounces of water could boost your metabolic rate by 30%. They further estimated that increasing water intake by 6 cups per day could lead to burning an extra 17,400 calories per year.

Health Promotion Practice posted a study online stating that receiving daily reminders to eat healthy and motivational tips helped people stick to healthy eating.

A study out of Tufts University found that people who had 3 servings of whole grains (oats, quinoa, wheat, etc) had 10% less abdominal fat than those who had 3 servings of refined carbs.

A recent study on a Mediterranean diet that included 2 servings of dark chocolate over one that didn't found that the chocolate infused diet resulted in better health.

Multiple studies suggest that exercising in the morning puts people in the healthy mindset and they will make healthier eating decisions throughout the day.

Shop seasonally. People are concerned that healthier food is more expensive. Eating seasonally can greatly reduce costs.

Month 9 Checklist

1. I am eating healthy lunch and dinners 6 out of 7 days a week ☐

Write down some new foods you want to try and some strategies on how to eat healthier moving forward.

# Month 10: Cardio

*Goal: 30 minutes per day, every day.  Develop a cardio routine.*

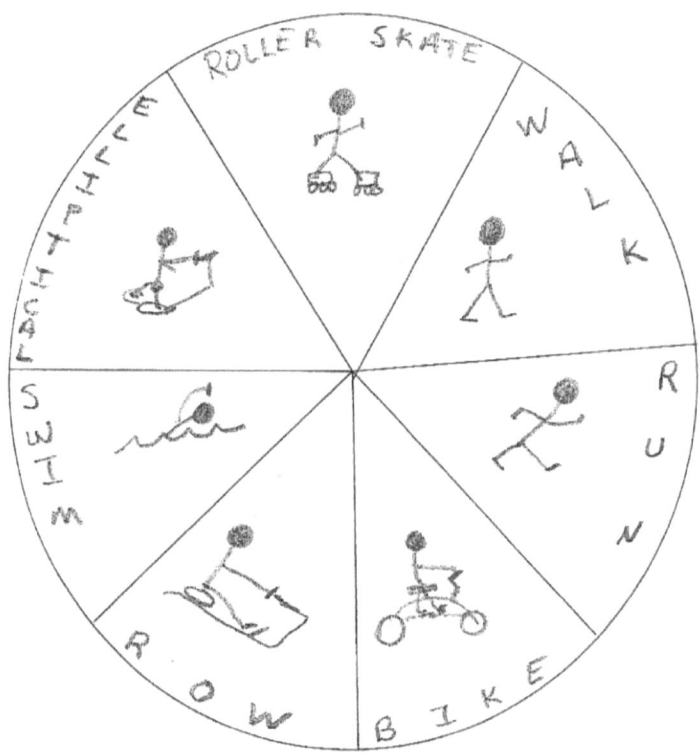

The goals are getting tougher.  This time you are not only upping your daily dose of cardio, but you are also learning to plan your workouts ahead.  This does not have to be anything complicated or convoluted.  Keep it simple.  So many people want to be professional athletes and come up with these insanely specific workouts.

*Ex.  20 min bike at 75% VO₂Max, 5 min at 90%, 5 min at 50%.*

You will spend ¾ of the time checking your pulse and figuring out needless equations.  Unless you are training and trying to get every last ounce of benefit in order to improve performance by minuscule numbers, then just do something challenging.

> My example for you:
> 20 min bike at intensity to get you breathing moderately well
> 5 min of biking at top speed
> 5 min of very light biking to relax
> End of work out—feel tired, heart rate is up, sweating

Yes, training in target heart rate zones and monitoring your % of VO$_2$Max (the amount of oxygen you can use) is important for performance based training and can be useful for health based training, but is certainly not necessary. I think the *tired rule* works just fine. If, at the end of the work out you are really tired, then you have probably done enough to get some benefit out of it. If you get to the end of the workout and feel that you could go on for 3 more hours, your workout has not been hard enough and you need to increase the intensity next time.

*Reminders on How to Workout*

A suggestion about "How" to perform your cardio is to keep it variable. Keep it variable in the workout and between workouts. In the workout, go hard for 5 minutes, tone it down for 5 minutes, ramp it up to a moderate intensity, then bring it back down. It forces your body to constantly adapt and adjust to changing needs (similar to real life). A lot of the new research I have been reading is showing very positive effects of interval training. Between workouts change it up. On Monday bike for 30 minutes at a constant/moderate rate. When you bike again on Wednesday, sprint the first 10 seconds of every minute, then relax for 50 seconds. In addition to challenging your body, it also helps change up the workouts over time (they can get monotonous real quick if you, are not careful). Remember there are many ways to get your cardio exercise in.

The last "How" topic before jumping into how to organize your schedule is overload. It is one of the most common principles in exercise prescription and can be applied to all types of exercise. As explained earlier, it means you have to continuously make things more difficult. For example, if you use the sprinting the first 10 seconds of every minute example, after you have done this a while, it will get easier and easier until you are not getting significant benefits from the workout anymore. If you continue to stay at that level, you will never improve, only maintain. To make this harder try sprinting 15 seconds or upping the intensity of the 50 second slow time. Always make your work out harder and more challenging if you want to continue to improve.

*Reminder on Organization*

How do we fit this in to our crazy schedule? An important rule to remember is that the ACSM and AHA both state that you need 30 minutes of moderate physical activity every day. The important part of this rule is that you can do 10 or 15 minutes at a time which makes squeezing it into your day easier. Go for a quick jog before your morning shower and a quick jog right after you get home. If you are fortunate enough to have a good lunch break, and even equipment at your disposal, work out at lunch! Other people need to get it all done in one shot. My personal preference is running in the morning before I have the whole day to convince myself I do not really have to do it after work. For right now, try and get in to a normal routine. Once you have established a routine and start getting bored with it, this is when you should think about changing it up.

Many people will start as, and even become, a weekend-warrior. These are the people that do nothing active all week and then try and do a week's worth of exercise in 2 days. I will save you the trouble and tell you it does NOT work. A lot of people get injured doing this because they over-train past fatigue on these days. Muscle strains and pains are common with these types of workouts. A better idea is to do something every day to build strength and endurance.

*A usual day for me*

*Run before work*
*Weights over lunch*
*Stretching/core training after work.*

It works best for me to split everything up. I have also found that working out in the middle of the workday really splits things up nicely and gives me a little boost for the afternoon.

When are your favorite times to do cardio?

1. _____
2. _____
3. _____
4. _____
5. _____

When are some realistic times for you to fit it in?

1. _____
2. _____
3. _____
4. _____
5. _____

What are some ways you can vary your workouts?

1. _____
2. _____
3. _____
4. _____
5. _____

**Here is a Cardio table. Fill in your daily activities. Fill in the activity and the amount of time.**

| Mon | Tues | Wed | Thurs | Fri | Sat | Sun |
|------|------|------|-------|------|------|------|
| Bike (35) | Run (20) | Run (25) | Bike (30) | Walk (60) | Row (40) | Walk (60) |
|  |  |  |  |  |  |  |
|  |  |  |  |  |  |  |

| | | | | | | |
|---|---|---|---|---|---|---|
| | | | | | | |
| | | | | | | |
| | | | | | | |
| | | | | | | |
| | | | | | | |

I mentioned VO$_2$Max earlier. As the intensity of your exercise goes up, so does the amount of oxygen you take in. At some point you reach a maximum where you can work out harder and harder, but the amount of oxygen you take in and use will not increase. This signifies the maximum amount of oxygen your body can take in to be used.

Why is this important? For those of you who are concerned about exercising in a target heart rate zone, knowing your VO$_2$Max can be very useful. A target heart rate zone is a range of your heart rate or VO$_2$Max that you try and work out in. It is an objective way of gauging how hard you are working out. The easiest way is to use your heart rate. A safe way to use your heart rate as a gauge is with the Karvonen formula:

**Target Heart Rate = ((max HR − resting HR) × %Intensity) + resting HR**

You will use this equation twice, once for the lower end of intensity and once for the upper end. The intensity in which you choose to work out is totally up to you. Anywhere from 60-80% is a good average zone.

The other option is to exercise based on a percentage of your $VO_2Max$. This requires far more knowledge and usually some equipment to make it more accurate—way above what is needed for the people reading this book.

*Research Recap*

Cardiovascular benefits are seen during high-paced strength training, particularly when less than 20 seconds is taken between sets.

Interval training can ramp up the intensity and calories burned. Interval training and things like Tabata are high intensity workouts that can provide better results in 10 minutes than some other hour-long programs.

Doing other exercises during "rest" breaks can significantly increase burned calories during an exercise session.

Training the arms is important even when most traditional cardio exercises focus on the legs. Improving the capacity of the arms can greatly improve your times and ability.

Researchers at the Cooper Institute for Aerobics Research in Dallas, Texas examined the effect of cardiorespiratory fitness on all-cause mortality and reported in the American Journal of Clinical Nutrition that lean men with low cardiorespiratory fitness were twice as likely to die from all causes than lean, cardio-fit men.

The Journal of Psychopharmacology reported that cardiorespiratory fitness is an indicator off all-cause cardiovascular disease mortality.

Mayo Clinic Proceedings reported that a lack of fitness elicits adverse metabolic changes that can lead to type 2 diabetes.

The Mayo Clinic Proceedings noted that there was a 64% decrease in the risk of heart disease in those that were aerobically fit vs. those who were not.

The CDC reported that performing moderately intensive aerobic exercise (jogging, weightlifting, etc) for 130-150 minutes/week can help avoid bone complications such as fractures and osteoporosis.

Month 10 Checklist

1. I am performing at least 30 minutes of cardio every day ☐

2. I enjoy the type of cardio exercise I am currently doing ☐

# Month 11: Resistance

*Goal: By the end of the month you will do resistance training at least 30 minutes per day, every day of the week.*

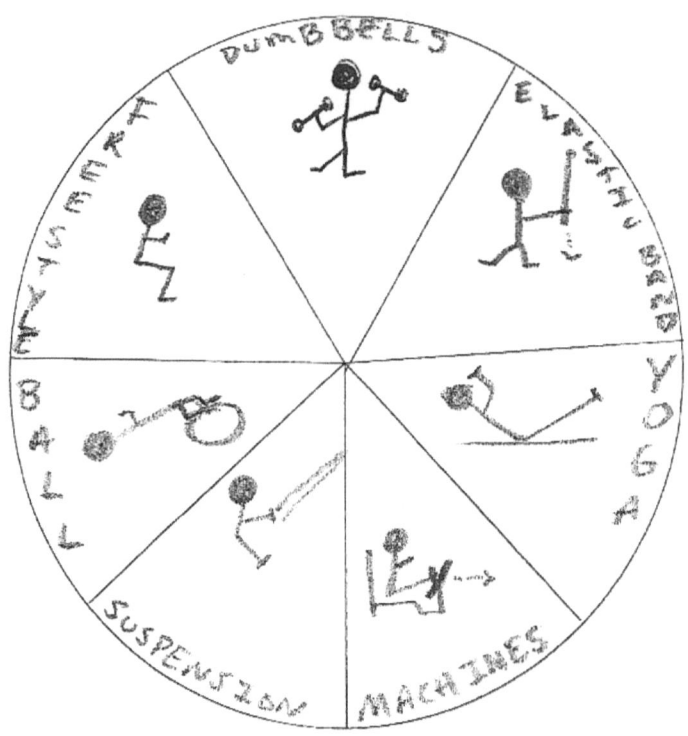

We have already discussed the role of the muscles and nerves in building your strength and the many other health benefits. This chapter is aimed at improving your resistance training routine and extending it to 7 days per week. We want to add variety to your workout to improve it and keep it interesting.

The last time we discussed resistance training was in the 5th month of your transformation. At this point you are performing resistance training 3 times per week for a total of 30 minutes each of those days. Most people at this point have a normal routine they follow (Tuesday/Thursday→Arms, Saturday→Core/legs. All with machines). The pie chart from the previous page is just to remind you that there are many ways of getting the necessary resistance training. If you are bored with your current routine, now is the time to start introducing new activities gradually.

This week you should try and do 5 days of resistance training. Try 3 days with your normal routine and change it up for the 4$^{th}$ and 5$^{th}$ days in the week. OR Normal routine/change/normal routine/change/normal routine.

Sometimes, there are constraints on how much variation there can be because of time, money, etc. Within each type of training, there are different ways to perform activities.

One way is to change the pace. This can be used with elastic bands, suspension system, dumbbells, machines, and freestyle! Most people perform 3 sets of 10 reps at the same pace, for every exercise, every time. The down side is that your body gets very efficient at this type of work and it becomes less of a challenge for the working muscles. Try the same exercises, but in one direction slow down significantly. Take the bicep curls. Curl up the weight at the same pace you always have. Now on the way down, go reaaaallllyyyy slow. Do this for every repetition. Warning—you might be a little sore and tired the next day. At the gym, people refer to these as "negatives" or "eccentrics". Whatever you call them, they are a great way to build muscle once you have built a good foundation of strength (as you already have after month 5!).

Plyometrics are a different form of resistance training that involves explosive movements.

These are only to be performed by people with a solid base of strength and are not for everyone. If you know a physical therapist, strength and conditioning specialist, or trainer, it would be advisable to consult with them to make sure you are prepared for plyometric training.

Plyometric exercises involve a quick stretch to the muscle and an immediate full force contraction (called the stretch-shortening cycle). This type of exercise increases the nervous system involvement and recruits more motor units in the muscle to create a stronger contraction in the muscle. Most of these exercises involve some kind of jumping motion. The number of repetitions/session varies among sources. Most recommendations I have seen for novices state 60 contractions/session, with up to 150 contractions/session for advanced athletes. My suggestion is to start very slow. These are very difficult and hard on your body. I tell people to start with 10. Wait 2 days and see how those muscles feel. If your muscles are still sore, stick with 10 until the pain stops after workouts. Once you can do 10 without any symptoms a couple days later, bump it to 20 and so on. Plyometrics can be performed by all ages if done correctly. My suggestion is to get some professional guidance to learn how to properly perform these exercises.

Who are some professionals in your area that could help you?
1. _____ Phone #_____
2. _____ Phone #_____
3. _____ Phone #_____
4. _____ Phone #_____
5. _____ Phone #_____

Most people think Olympic lifting is only for the seasoned veteran. To do it like the professionals, this is true. But most of us are not professionals and we still want different ways to get stronger. Olympic lifting is basically two movements: the snatch and the clean-and-jerk. The snatch is where the exerciser lifts the bar from the ground straight overhead in one fluid motion landing in the squat position. The clean is where the bar is picked up from the ground onto the person's shoulders. The jerk is where the bar is lifted overhead and the person ends in the lunge position (one foot bent in front of the other). Both motions require full-body participation and are therefore fantastic exercises to perform. My suggestion is to seek professional help initially to focus solely on form. You want to be able to perform both of these movements holding an un-weighted bar with perfect form before ever thinking about adding weights. Be careful, most trainers want to add weight right away. Trust me, become a perfectionist about form.

When you have done that, start adding weight and you will reap the benefits.

Suspension bands are a new variation in the exercise world. They take advantage of your body weight for resistance. The anchor is hung over a door or in a tree and you hold on to handles at the end of 2 bands. Upper body, core, and lower body exercises can be performed with these bands. Where and/or how you decide to stand will affect the resistance you will work against. These are an easy way for beginners to get started. For $50 you can get a set of bands and a small instructional booklet to help get you started (deluxe versions start around $100) without any other equipment. They really are a great deal and are a great way to vary your exercise program.

Kettle bells are the new craze. They are essentially medicine balls with a handle. Anyone can perform simple kettle bell exercises. The most important thing to do is to perform these activities with proper form. Most of the movements require a swinging motion that requires all of your trunk muscles to be activated to maintain stability through the whole motion. If done correctly, these are great whole body workouts.

What are some exercises out there that you have not tried?
1. _____
2. _____
3. _____
4. _____
5. _____

What are some exercises out there that you want to try?
1. _____
2. _____
3. _____

**Fill out the table below throughout this month.**

| Date | Total Time | Activity | Feelings |
|------|-----------|----------|----------|
| 4-30-11 | 45 (all AM) | Suspension bands | Great change of pace |
| 5-2-11 | 30 (AM/PM) | Olympic lifting | Too intense for me |
| | | | |
| | | | |
| | | | |
| | | | |
| | | | |
| | | | |
| | | | |

|  |  |  |  |
|---|---|---|---|
|  |  |  |  |
|  |  |  |  |
|  |  |  |  |
|  |  |  |  |
|  |  |  |  |
|  |  |  |  |
|  |  |  |  |
|  |  |  |  |
|  |  |  |  |

|  |  |  |  |
|---|---|---|---|
|  |  |  |  |
|  |  |  |  |
|  |  |  |  |
|  |  |  |  |
|  |  |  |  |
|  |  |  |  |
|  |  |  |  |

*Research Recap*

Tufts University reported on a strength-training program with older men and women with moderate to severe knee arthritis. The results of this sixteen-week program showed that strength training decreased pain by 43%, increased muscle strength and general physical performance, improved the clinical signs and symptoms of the disease, and decreased disability. The effectiveness of strength training to ease the pain of arthritis was just as potent, if not more potent, as medications. Similar effects of strength training have been seen in patients with rheumatoid arthritis.

The CDC reports that as people age, poor balance and flexibility contribute to falls and broken bones. These fractures can result in significant disability and, in some cases, death. Strengthening exercises, when done properly and through the full range of motion, increase a person's flexibility and balance, which decrease the likelihood and severity of falls.

A study in New Zealand in women 80 years of age and older showed a 40% reduction in falls with simple strength and balance training.

Post-menopausal women can lose 1-2% of their bone mass annually. Results from a study conducted at Tufts University, which were published in the *Journal of the American Medical Association* in 1994, showed that strength training increases bone density and reduces the risk for fractures among women aged 50-70.

Strength training is crucial to weight control, because individuals who have more muscle mass have a higher metabolic rate. Muscle is active tissue that consumes calories while stored fat uses very little energy. Strength training can provide up to a 15% increase in metabolic rate, which is enormously helpful for weight loss and long-term weight control.

More than 14 million Americans have type II diabetes—a staggering three hundred percent increase over the past forty years—and the numbers are steadily climbing. In addition to being at greater risk for heart and renal disease, diabetes is also the leading cause of blindness in older adults. Fortunately, studies now show that lifestyle changes such as strength training have a profound impact on helping older adults manage their diabetes. In a recent study of Hispanic men and women, 16 weeks of strength training produced dramatic improvements in glucose control that are comparable to taking diabetes medication. Additionally, the study volunteers were stronger, gained muscle, lost body fat, had less depression, and felt much more self-confident.

Strength training provides similar improvements in depression as anti-depressant medications. Currently, it is not known if this is because people feel better when they are stronger or if strength training produces a helpful biochemical change in the brain. It is most likely a combination of the two. When older adults participate in strength training programs, their self-confidence and self-esteem improve, which has a strong impact on their overall quality of life.

Scientific research has shown that exercise can slow the physiological aging clock. While aerobic exercise, such as walking, jogging, or swimming, has many excellent health benefits—it maintains the heart and lungs and increases cardiovascular fitness and endurance—it does not make your muscles strong. Strength training does. Studies have shown that lifting weights two or three times a week increases strength by building muscle mass and bone density.

One 12-month study conducted on postmenopausal women at Tufts University demonstrated 1% gains in hip and spine bone density, 75% increases in strength and 13% increases in dynamic balance with just two days per week of progressive strength training. The control group had losses in bone, strength, and balance. Strength training programs can also have a profound effect on reducing risk for falls, which translates to fewer fractures.

Month 11 Checklist

1. I am performing at least 30 minutes of resistance training every day ☐

2. I enjoy the type of resistance training I am currently doing ☐

# Month 12: Wrapping it Up

*Goal: Assess what you have done so far, look for potential pitfalls, adjust routines, etc. Move Forward! Keep Going!*

It is time for me to wrap things up. Over the next month you will need to finalize your workout routine and secure the continuation of your new lifestyle. We have a few major categories: Planning, Motivation, Diet, Cardio, Resistance, and Flexibility.

Your planning has been a significant portion of your journey as the major topic in 2 full months and a large part of this chapter. It is such a crucial part of the lifestyle improvement and is always ignored (which is why I have drawn so much attention to it). At this point, you should be a member of a gym and/or have the necessary equipment to perform activities at home. You should have a calendar to help organize all of these new additions and activities. Your exercise and diet should fit smoothly and seamlessly into your new life.

Motivation goes right along with planning as underappreciated when developing a healthy lifestyle change (or poorly organized, set up for failure). Use something that works for you. Remember to change it up if your current form of motivation is not working for you. Be proud of what you have accomplished. Be excited about your potential for further improvement.

Healthy diet can transform your life. It can affect your energy levels, make you feel good, help you lose weight, and become healthier (among so many other benefits). We have talked a lot about your diet and some specifics about why you choose certain foods and not others. At this point in the program, you should be eating healthy all the time. Remember though, it is OK to splurge occasionally. Research shows that it is good for you mentally and behaviorally to eat differently sometimes. Going out to eat at a restaurant twice in a month is great! Eat, drink, and be merry. The problem starts when this becomes a staple of your normal diet. Eat in moderation. Eat a varied and colorful diet.

Cardiovascular exercise might be the single most important thing you can do for yourself. It does not tend to be a fan favorite, but it could not be more important to your health and longevity. Performing daily cardiovascular exercise will transform your life for the better.

Resistance training is usually peoples' "go-to move" when beginning exercise. This is partially because no one likes cardio and partially because everyone thinks they can just lift a few weights and create a smokin' bod. Remember to be creative with your routine. If you get done with a workout and you are not tired and thought it was easy, so did your body. You need to make it harder—increase the weight/reps or even the activities you are doing. Always challenge your body to adapt. Always challenge your body to do more.

 We have covered every topic you need to succeed in this lifestyle change. As you come to the last few pages of this book, what are some areas that you feel need some fine-tuning this last month? Do you see any potential roadblocks?

1. _____
2. _____
3. _____
4. _____
5. _____

Before making any new changes to your program, address these. These small problems can become a hassle. This program should run smoothly and efficiently.

Once you have addressed these, start thinking about new goals for yourself. At this point in the program, you want to make long-term goals for yourself. Where do you want to be in 6, 12, 24 months? What are some things you can work towards? In 12 months, would you like to run a marathon? Finish a triathlon?

What are some long-term goals?
1. _____
2. _____
3. _____
4. _____
5. _____

General Goals

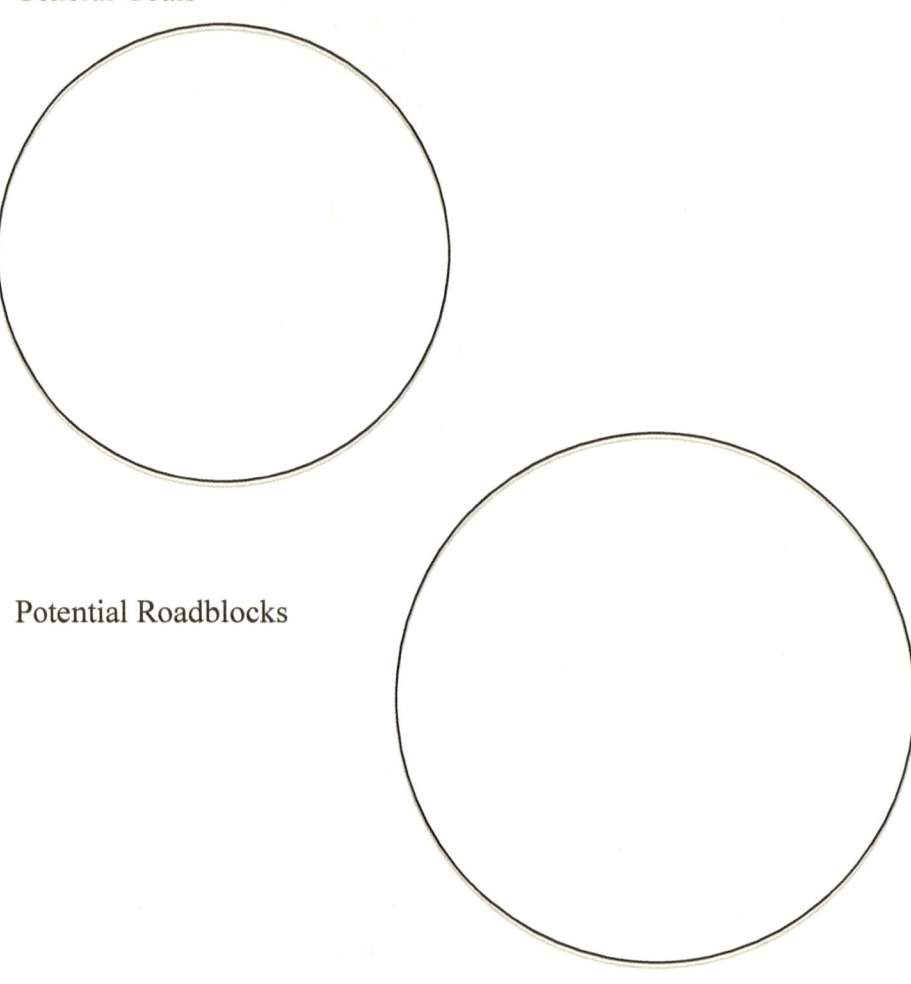

Potential Roadblocks

Solutions

## Month 12 Checklist

1. I have proper workout clothing/shoes for all activities I will be performing…☐
2. I have a gym membership or all of the necessary equipment to carry out my daily activity routine…☐
3. I have a safe place at home or to go to exercise…☐
4. I have a local supermarket(s) that carry the foods I will need to maintain a healthy and varied diet…☐
5. I have a system in place to make sure I will eat healthily every day…☐
6. I have allotted time in my daily life to allow for at least 30 minutes of resistance training, 30 minutes of cardiovascular training, and flexibility on the required days…☐
7. I have a large calendar to help organize my day around getting healthy…☐
8. I have a journal to record my diet and exercise for each day…☐

**Insert a picture of yourself.**

Take a moment to write down anything you have accomplished.
Admire what a successful year you have had and keep going!

## VOCABULARY

**Concentric contraction**: shortening the muscle against resistance. It would be the phase of a biceps curl where you are pulling the weight up. The phase where you lower it is considered eccentric (muscle lengthening against resistance).

**Cardiopulmonary System**: consists of your heart and lungs. It is responsible with getting rid of waste products (mainly $CO_2$), replenishing blood with oxygen, and pumping the blood out to the wanting tissue.

**Cardiovascular System**: consists of all the heart and vessels in the body. It is responsible for transporting blood all over the body.

**Eccentrics (Negatives):** a weightlifting technique where you add resistance as the muscle is lengthening. An example would be lowering a biceps curl very slowly back down to your side. The phase where you lift the biceps curl up is considered a concentric contraction because the muscle is shortening.

**VO$_2$Max**: in short, the maximum volume of $O_2$ your body can consume and use.

## Before and After

I thought it was only fair that I included a picture of me before and after I completed my own program. I lost a 30 pounds and have never felt better!

**Zazzle.com/SmartLife**

Check out all the great Smart Life products!

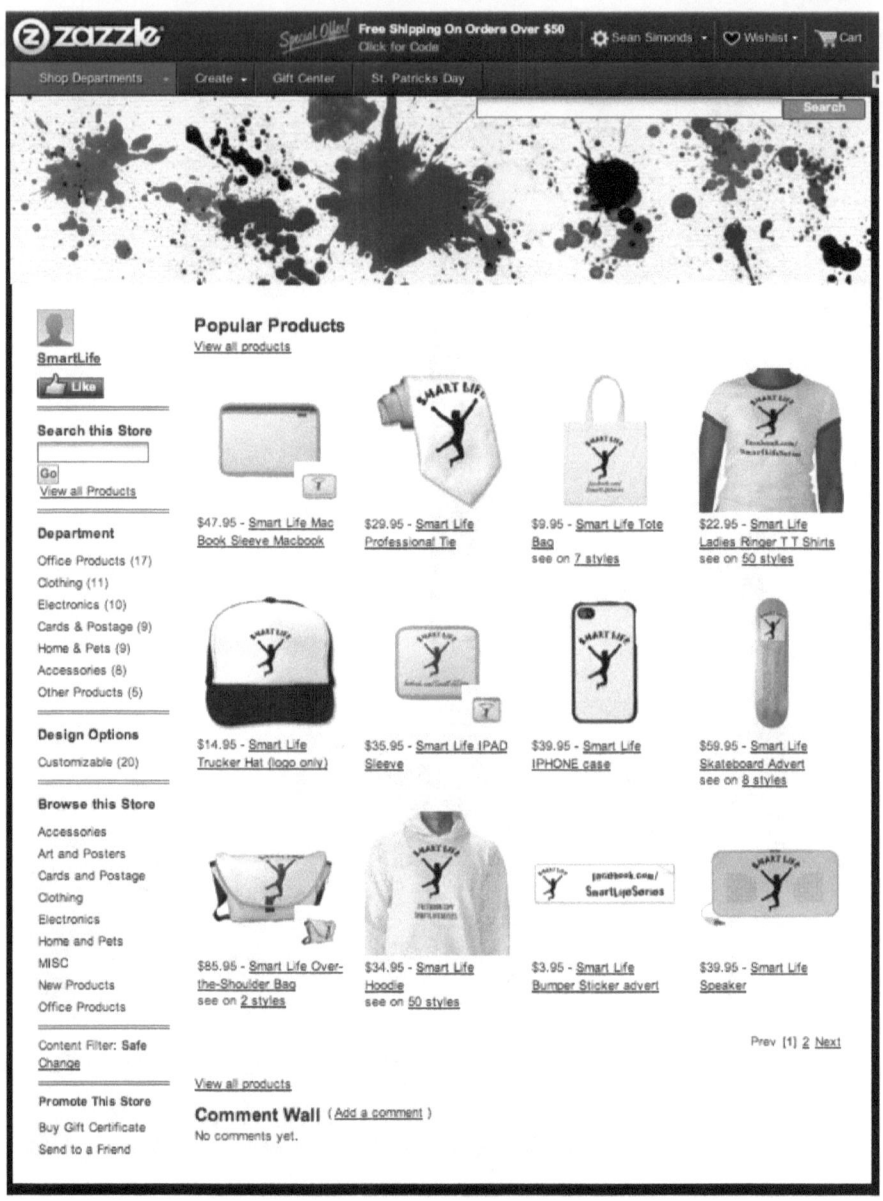

# www.TheSmartLifeSeries.com

Check the website for extra free information, videos, etc.!
Follow the blog at: www.TheSmartLifeSeries.com/Smart-Life

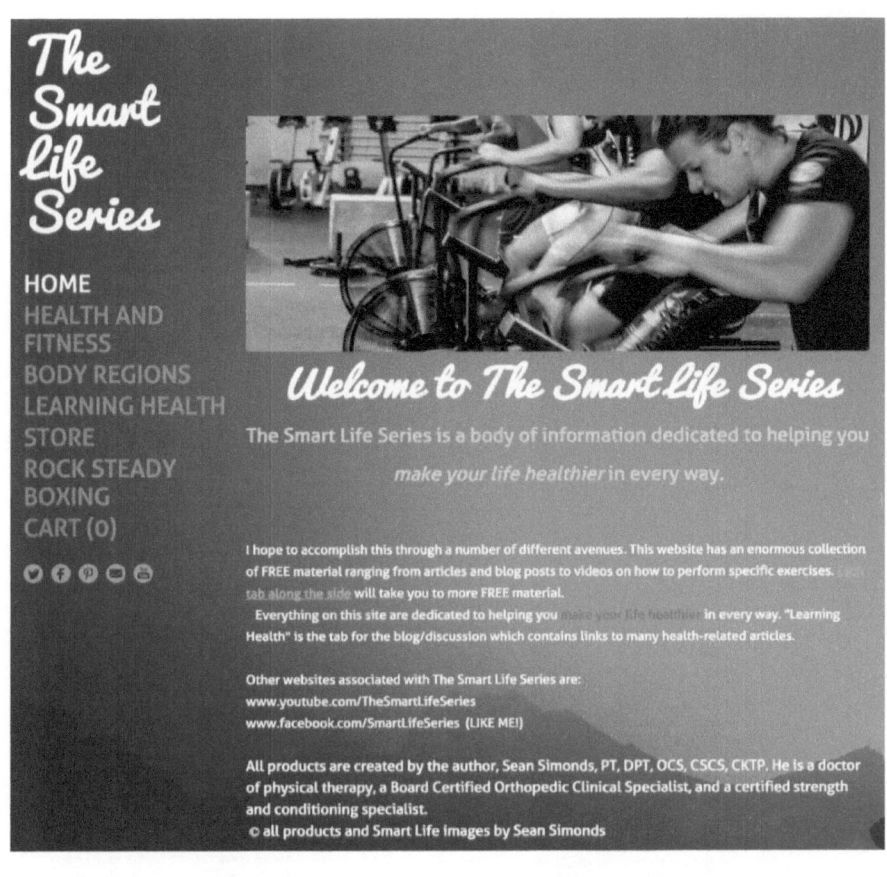

**The Smart Life Series**

HOME
HEALTH AND FITNESS
BODY REGIONS
LEARNING HEALTH
STORE
ROCK STEADY BOXING
CART (0)

**Welcome to The Smart Life Series**

The Smart Life Series is a body of information dedicated to helping you *make your life healthier* in every way.

I hope to accomplish this through a number of different avenues. This website has an enormous collection of FREE material ranging from articles and blog posts to videos on how to perform specific exercises. Each tab along the side will take you to more FREE material.

Everything on this site are dedicated to helping you make your life healthier in every way. "Learning Health" is the tab for the blog/discussion which contains links to many health-related articles.

Other websites associated with The Smart Life Series are:
www.youtube.com/TheSmartLifeSeries
www.facebook.com/SmartLifeSeries (LIKE ME!)

All products are created by the author, Sean Simonds, PT, DPT, OCS, CSCS, CKTP. He is a doctor of physical therapy, a Board Certified Orthopedic Clinical Specialist, and a certified strength and conditioning specialist.
© all products and Smart Life images by Sean Simonds

**"Like" us at: Facebook.com/SmartLifeSeries**
Come and check out all the new information and updates!

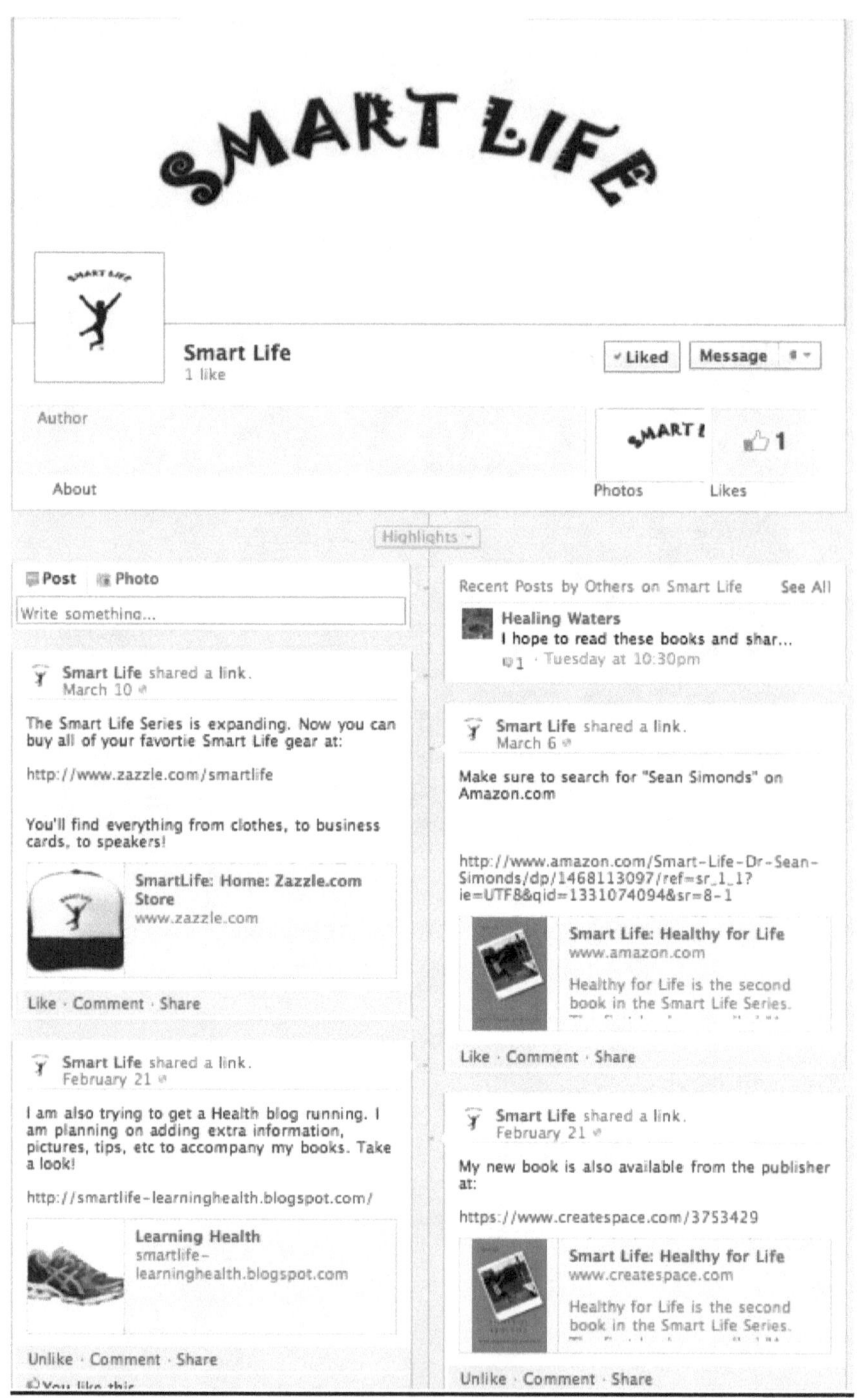

## References

1. Mayo Clinic Online at www.Mayoclinic.com
2. American Heart Association at www.heart.org
3. Smart Life/Learning Health Blog at http://smartlife-learninghealth.blogspot.com/
4. USDA at www.usda.gov
5. Magee, David. Orthopedic Physical Assessment. Saunders. 5th Ed. 2007
6. Dutton, Mark. Orthopedic Examination, Evaluation, and Intervention. McGraw Hill Medical. 2nd Ed. 2008
7. Goodman, C. Pathology: Implications for the Physical Therapist. Suanders. 3rd Ed. 2006
8. O'sullivan, S. Physical Rehabilitation. F.A. Davis Company. 5th Ed. 2006
9. www.EatThis.com
10. Franklin, B. and McCullough, P. Cardiorespiratory Fitness: An Independent and Additive Marker of Risk Stratification and Health Outcomes. Mayo Clinic Proceedings. 2009
11. http://www.cdc.gov/physicalactivity/growingstronger/why/

www.ingramcontent.com/pod-product-compliance
Lightning Source LLC
Chambersburg PA
CBHW050448290526
45786CB00006B/2206